THE ALKALINE FIX

HEAL YOUR BODY AND RECLAIM YOUR HEALTH WITH THE POWER OF THE ALKALINE DIET

Lauren Clark

© Copyright 2019 – All rights reserved.

This document is geared towards providing exact and reliable information in regards to the topic and issue covered. The publication is sold with the idea that the publisher is not required to render accounting, officially permitted, or otherwise, qualified services. If advice is necessary, legal or professional, a practiced individual in the profession should be ordered.

From a Declaration of Principles which was accepted and approved equally by a Committee of the American Bar Association and a Committee of Publishers and Associations.

In no way is it legal to reproduce, duplicate, or transmit any part of this document in either electronic means or in printed format. Recording of this publication is strictly prohibited and any storage of this document is not allowed unless with written permission from the publisher. All rights reserved.

The information provided herein is stated to be truthful and consistent, in that any liability, in terms of inattention or otherwise, by any usage or abuse of any policies, processes, or directions contained within is the solitary and utter responsibility of the recipient reader. Under no circumstances will any legal responsibility or blame be held against the publisher for any reparation, damages, or monetary loss due to the information herein, either directly or indirectly.

The information herein is offered for informational purposes solely and is universal as so. The presentation of the information is without a contract or any type of guarantee assurance.

The trademarks that are used are without any consent, and the publication of the trademark is without permission or backing by the trademark owner. All trademarks and brands within this book are for clarifying purposes only and are owned by the owners themselves, not affiliated with this document.

ABOUT LAUREN CLARK

FEELING GOOD SHOULDN'T BE COMPLICATED – IT'S JUST MADE TO SEEM THAT WAY.

The World Health Organization (WHO) defines health as a state of complete physical, mental, and social well-being and not merely the absence of disease or infirmity.

The formula is simple: enough movement, plenty of whole foods, awareness of your body, and adapting the right mindset, are the keys to a healthy and happy life. While calorie restriction can seem effective, depriving your body of proper nutrition isn't sustainable. Neither is it healthy for your body or mind – especially when you get caught in a dieting cycle.

Lauren Clark hopes to change the conversation. she helps people build long-term healthy habits in a way that doesn't feel limiting, but instead empowering and enjoyable.

Lauren Clark is a health and wellness enthusiast and author of The Acid Reflux Fix and other health and wellness related books. Having struggled with gut health and eating disorders from a young age, Lauren has always searched for natural cures and remedies because she believes that mother nature always has the answers if we look hard enough.

Now, Lauren is dedicated to raising awareness of the importance of living a healthy life and helping people just like you regain what matters: their physical and mental health. After all, the journey to optimal health should be celebrated.

CONTENTS

INTRODUCTION

For you to have this book, you must be in search of freedom from "food rules" and obviously, you are curious about how to achieve optimum health. This book is here to provide more than you can ask for or think of. Achieving optimum health is made easy; let's take you on a ride.

Achieving optimum health isn't a tough walk to freedom; rather, it is all about the right knowledge. It is an array of well-defined steps with flexibility, but how would you know? This book is, therefore, written to enlighten you, but the right knowledge is empowerment.

To remain healthy, the kind of food you eat means a whole lot. Particularly these days that we are altogether encompassed by compulsions to eat excessively, and a lot of the wrong thing.

How would you be able ever to envision that health isn't significant?

If you don't have your health, what do you have? If you are weak and tired constantly and your body won't do what you need it to, suppose that you are in pains constantly, what good is anything else? Regardless of whether you earn all the cash on the planet, of what good is wealth without health?

As indicated by the World Health Organization (WHO), Health is characterized as: "A state of optimal well-being, not merely the absence of disease and infirmity."

Health is a major and key pre-imperative for us to live our lives. Health resembles a vehicle, and the Life resembles a trip in it. To begin the vehicle and push it forward, the vehicle must be in a decent condition. In like manner, to begin the life and live it to the fullest, health is unavoidably a necessity.

Have you at any point thought about whether a significant number of the illnesses seething through our general public have a common reason? Do you sit and imagine the source of most diseases? Aren't you marveled and most times perplex as to what is healthy and what isn't?

Over acidity, which can turn into a risky condition that debilitates all body's frameworks, is common today. It makes the internal environment conducive for sickness, rather than a pH-balanced state which helps the body to oppose illness. It is the start of all problems with health and the body. As we know that all diseases and infections find their start point from the gut, which is where the first contact comes. It is essential to know and keep what goes into the gut as healthy as possible.

A healthy body keeps up sufficient alkaline stores to meet demands. At the point when excess acids must be neutralized, our alkaline stores are depleted, leaving the body in a weakened condition. An Acid Alkaline Balanced diet is a crucial key to health upkeep.

The food we eat enters the body's cells and is utilized to support the cells. Along these lines, toxins can enter as well and damage the cells. An aggregation of these squanders and toxins make the cells age and at times makes it change to a wiped out or irregular cell. Long periods of collection of this toxic slime in tissues and cells can prompt poor blood and lymph circulation, even poor cell action. Therefore, results in the counteractive action of supplements from entering the cells, a debilitating of the cells that finally lead to sicknesses. It is currently evident that this toxic slime is the fundamental reason for health conditions, for example, heart maladies, malignancy, joint pain and gout, weight, kidney ailments, diabetes, to refer to yet a couple.

Imagine a portion of the food you routinely long for: pizza, hamburger, steak, processed meals, etc. Obviously, these things are delicious; however, meat and carb-substantial food you've become used to might put you in danger for chronic sicknesses. What's more, the purpose behind that may come down to this: acid-alkaline imbalance.

The pH (capability of hydrogen) scale estimates precisely how acidic or how soluble a solution is. It ranges from 0 to 14, where the lower the pH, the more acidic, and the higher the pH, the more alkaline. What's more, when a solution is totally nonpartisan, similar to water, it has a pH of 7.

To survive your blood must keep up an exceptionally sensitive pH parity scope of 7.35 to 7.45. Whenever a pH lopsidedness happens and results in acidic blood that is out of this range, the blood ends up unfit to convey sufficient oxygen and shield the body from infection. Fortunately, your body is supported with a few control instruments that help manage your pH and shield you from falling into this threat zone, but your body can turn out to be less productive if you continue filling it with the wrong sort of fuel, which in your body's case is food.

Each sort of food has its own pH. A few foods, for example, avocado and quinoa, are alkalizing and have an alkaline effect on the body. Different foods, like most meats and dairy, are acidifying and make it increasingly hard for the body to work.

The stomach is acidic, with a pH of 3.5 or beneath, so it experiences no difficulty separating antacid foods. Acidic foods are anything you expend with a pH under 7. A few examples of acidic foods are coffee, dairy products, sugar, prepared or restored meats and an assortment of different things.

It is expected that we eat at least 70% of alkaline-producing foods in our eating routine, to look after our health. We need a lot of fresh foods grown from the ground and to adjust our essential protein consumption. What's more, we have to stay away from prepared, sugary, or processed foods, since they are acidic as well as they raise glucose level too rapidly. Besides, they will be in general supplements lacking in nutrition and might be harmful as well.

Furthermore, imagine a scenario where you are trying to achieve optimum health through restrictive dieting. Imagine that you have been denying yourself horribly and are attempting to come back to a progressively adjusted methodology. All that weight is no assistance to you either. Obviously, you have to take handy measures to deal with your food consumption and set up a decent daily schedule; however, you will be significantly more prone to get tired of the whole process. But with the help of this book, a distinctive and straightforward assistance, less effort will yield enough results.

The way to health is not in compulsive dieting and impossible diet routines. The acid-alkaline balance is one of the best ways forward and will be discussed in detail in this book.

In this book, you will find handy information that has been exquisitely crafted in an informative yet beginner-friendly way to help you achieve optimum health through acid-alkaline balance. It emphasizes the importance of loving yourself and nurturing yourself through the process of balancing acidity and alkalinity in your body.

Are you prepared to peruse the first part? Just keep flipping through the pages.

DISCLAIMER

The author of this book is not a physician, and the ideas, procedures, and suggestions in this book are not intended as a substitute for the medical advice of a trained health professional. All matters regarding your health require medical supervision. Consult your doctor before adopting the suggestions in this book

This book was written for educational purposes only.

The author and publisher disclaim any liability arising directly or indirectly from the use of the book, or of any products mentioned herein.

Happy Reading!

CHAPTER 01

WHAT IS pH AND WHY DOES IT MATTER?

Over the years, a lot of questions have emerged as relating to pHand what it actually means? I'm sure, for at least once in your life so far, you have wondered what pH stands for or where the term originated from? I'm pleased to tell you that in this book, I wouldn't just answer this question but also carefully explain mind bothering questions and give solutions to many of the problems you might be encountering.

pH DEFINED.

pH is simply the measure of how acidic or alkaline (basic) a water-soluble(aqueous) substance is. It is also the measure of the Hydrogen ion (H+) concentration of a solution. To explain this, solutions with high concentrations of hydrogen ion (H+) have low pH while solutions with low concentrations of hydrogen ion have high pH.

i.e. Low concentration of hydrogen ion = High pH

A high concentration of hydrogen ion = Low pH

It is important you know that pH is an acronym for 'potential of hydrogen' or 'power of hydrogen.' Where 'p' stands for the German word for power, which is 'potenz and H is the element symbol for 'Hydrogen.' Note that 'H' is capitalized because it is most appropriate to capitalize symbols and letters representing an element. (Can you recall a little of your basic chemistry?) This term/acronym was coined by a Danish Biochemist Søren Peter Lauritz Sørensen in 1909.

To measure pH, a pH scale that numbers from one to fourteen is employed. This pH scale is used to specify how acidic or basic a water-based solution is. Acidic solutions have a lower pH (i.e., they have a higher concentration of Hydrogen ions), while alkaline solutions have a higher pH with low Hydrogen ion concentration. The middle number on the scale is seven, which is tagged as neutral. Substances with the pH value of seven are neither acidic nor basic/alkaline. They are referred to as neutral.

In summary,

Lower pH = Acidic Solutions = high concentration of H+

High pH = Basic or Alkaline solutions = Low concentration of H+

An acid has pH values between one and six. The

higher the pH value, the less acidic the substance is. An example of an acidic substance is carbon dioxide – that natural air you breathe out all day. This points to the fact that there exist naturally occurring acids and alkaline substances in the body. A base is the polar opposite of an acid, having between pH value eight to fourteen. These bases that occur naturally in the body are known to help neutralize acidity. A prominent example of a base is an essential component of the human body tissue – Bicarbonate (HCO3).

OTHER BASES ARE

- CALCIUM

Calcium is stored in almost all parts of the body. It is found in your bones, teeth, and even in the cells. Calcium is a rich, alkaline source. Calcium has a pH of about 9-10. This element, calcium, is known as a pH buffer. It neutralizes acidity. The process by which it dies this is called leaching. Leeching is bad for your bones though great for your blood.

- POTASSIUM AND MAGNESIUM

Potassium and magnesium with about 9-10 pH value, when consumed and broken down within the body, they produce alkaline ash or alkaline residues. Potassium and Magnesium, together with calcium work in harmony to help control your muscles. The heart is a muscle. These nutrients are, therefore, essential to help you manage your heart rate.

Note that, Bicarbonate is released and controlled by the kidney as needed in the body. It is the body's primary alkaline source. Just as the work of bases is to neutralize acidity, bicarbonate helps achieve body acid-base balance.

Enough of the chemistry! I know you might be bored with all of my stories, but a little concept understood here, and there is what makes knowledge. In terms of excess base/alkaline level in the body, there are naturally occurring acids too that neutralizes the excess alkaline effect. And they include:

- HYDROCHLORIC ACID

This acid is found in the stomach. It is useful in the digestion of foods. The acid's pH is about 2.0 on the pH scale and therefore accounts for fits strong acidity. A more relevant illustration is when you have acid reflux (what you most times call heartburn). It is as a result of your stomach Hydrochloric acid that burbles up to your throat. It is most frequent when you eat too many acidic foods. It can, sometimes, be a symptom of stomach ulcer.

- LACTIC ACID

Lactic acid is perfectly described as an exhaust

pipe. Yucky yet important, lactic acid has a pH value of about 3.0. It is an acid produced when you use energy to move or carry out any activity. It can be tagged the byproduct of energy consumption during work.

- CARBONIC ACID

When you breathe out, it is carbonic acid that is expelled from your body system. I'm accurately sure you just exhaled or yawned in about a few seconds ago. Carbonic acid with the pH by-product of respiration/breathing. This process is marked as oxygen, is breath in; it fills the lung and after that transported to every cell in your body through the cells. The by-product/waste is returned to the lungs and then exhaled. This exhaled air is carbonic acid.

To digest food or inflate your lungs, to regulate your body temperature and filter blood or to do any of life's activities, your body always makes use of energy. And while these processes are going on, a byproduct is created – Acid. So as your body produces energy, it produces acids alongside.

Values on the pH scale, called the pH value, are numbers from one to fourteen. Logically, the midpoint of these numbers is the number seven; therefore, seven is considered as the neutral point on the scale. Values that are below seven that is from one to six are considered acidic, and this increases as the pH value decreases. While, pH values that exceed seven are alkaline and also increases with an increase in value. It is important to note and keep in mind that a solution must be aqueous, i.e. must be in a solution or fluid form to have a pH.

The sour flavor present in food is as a result of the free hydrogen ions present in acidic foods. So, in other words, pH is said to be the measure of the number of free Hydrogen ions present in an aqueous solution.

pH AND YOUR HEALTH

Did you know? That your body is composed of thousands of trillions of microscopic cells. Each cell (smallest unit of life/ a living thing) has a membrane that encloses its content, keeping its valuables intact and maintains a particular standard in the cell. This includes the pH. Collectively, your cells, in their groups, create your internal pH environment, and this is directly proportional to the overall amount of acids and bases throughout the body. Hence, all of your body functions, abilities, and activities are influenced by this. The body becomes accommodating to certain bacteria, viruses, yeasts, and harmful organisms when the body's pH is acidic. Therefore, balancing the pH is a very important and crucial step in attaining and achieving optimum health. You might have been inviting diseases and unfriendly visitors due to the kind of foods you eat. Henceforth, learn not to create an environment conducive for germs, infections, and diseases. This is why alkalizing foods are advised in the right proportion with the acidic food in order to stay healthy and strong.

As discussed earlier, with too much free Hydrogen ion in your body, you become too acidic. Likewise, a deficit in the appropriate amount of Hydrogen ion makes you too alkaline too. The perfect environment and pH for your body to function appropriately is that condition that is slightly alkaline. This is proven as most of the body fluids are designed slightly alkaline, i.e., the lymphatic fluid, cerebrospinal fluid, liver bile, etc. The only internal body fluid that isn't slightly alkaline is that of the stomach (Hydrochloric Acid). When the body is becoming acidic, these acids (free Hydrogen ions) look for alkaline materials to react with.

Aside from dietary sources of these alkaline minerals, alkaline reserves are found in the liver, ligaments, muscles, and bones. When alkaline minerals are too little in food, and cells produce acid as a by-product, the acids are recycled to produce carbon dioxide and water which are excreted, afterward, harmlessly.

LET'S DO AN UNVEILING! NOTE THESE

- Feeling tired, groggy, irritated easily

- Weight gain, even after dieting

- Stomach upset and frequent digestive

problems

- Unhealthy skin, nails, and hair or even hair loss

- Frequent illness

- Digestive Issues

- Excess stomach acid

- Acid reflux

- Gastritis

- Ulcers

- Weird taste of the saliva

- Cracks at the corners of the lips

- Hives

- Very pale face

- Teeth and Mouth Issues

- Loose teeth

- Teeth are too sensitive

- Teeth aches and crack

- Gums ache at every temperature of food, whether cold, warm or hot.

- Mouth ulcers

- Throat infections and Tonsils infection.

- Eyes, Head and General Body

- Headaches

- Low body temperature (feels cold)

- Leg cramps and spasms

- Low energy; constant fatigue

- Excessive nervousness

These and many more are signs that you're acidic. That is, you've been consuming a lot of acidic foods, and you do not have a balanced pH.

Oh! Wait! Did I just describe you? Stay calm and keep reading. This book isn't one that locates a problem without showing the solution. It is worth the read. Let's take you on a ride!

HOW THEN DO I KNOW MY pH LEVEL?

Actually, there is an exact pH necessary for the health of blood and cells, organs and external fluids, skin and hair. Your pH level varies slightly depending on which body fluid you test. There is an exact pH necessary for the health of blood, cells, organs, external fluids, skin and hair.

But your blood is the most sensitive to pH fluctuations and changes over time and diet type. The average pH levels for bodily fluids are:

- Tears = 7.20

- Blood = 7.41

- Urine = 6.5 - 8.0

- Sweat = < 6.0

The blood's standard pH is 7.41. It implies that the blood is slightly alkaline. Any change in this standard initiates a body-wide chain reaction where excess acids that are present in the bloodstream are transported out and disposed into your tissues. When the limit is reached or slightly exceeded in the tissues, acids are forwarded and excreted through your urine or sweat. This is to help return the blood pH to normality. On average, in a healthy person, the tissue pH ranges from 7.35-7.45, but your sweats are always acidic with about 6.0 pH value.

It is obvious from all of our talks now that pH measurement is an ever-changing one. It can keep fluctuating once not balanced and maintained. In fact, your pH measurement can vary throughout a particular day. So, when you talk about altering your pH through diet, you are not just altering the pH of your blood of tissue but the pH of your body as a whole.

In summary, blood pH can influence tissue pH, and tissue pH can influence the sweat and Urine pH The effect is on all and not just one. You should be happy then that the body's pH can change, if it weren't ever-changing, there could be no way you could fix your imbalance. But thank goodness, solutions abound for all of your worries!!!

WHAT IS YOUR pH BALANCE?

pH balance can be called acid-base balance or acid-alkaline balance. It is that particular level of acids and bases/alkaline minerals that your body needs to work most effectively. At pH balance, your body works at its best. The body was made to work effectively at a particular state and is also equipped to maintain that healthy balance between acidity/acridity and alkalinity or basicity. But with anomalies, there is certain disruption from the environment, our diet, diseases, etc.

Disruption in your pH balance can lead to numerous medical conditions, but these are majorly classified into two, namely:

- Acidosis

- Alkalosis

When certain symptoms present the possibility of you having pH imbalance, you must seek medical attention fast. Tests will be carried out by your doctor/physician to determine the cause of the imbalance.

Always remember that your pH is critical to your health. Once the cause is discovered, follow the prescribed guidelines to make sure your pH is balanced once more.

WHY SHOULD YOU TEST YOUR BODY'S pH?

pH testing helps you to know

- When something goes wrong from the usual in your body.

- The presence of any disease or infections that can alter the pH balance.

- How well you are managing your body's pH and health as a whole.

- When to take immediate actions towards the balance of your health.

TESTING THE PH LEVELS OF THE BODY

To remain healthy, the slightly alkaline level of the body, which is the norm must be maintained. This is not nullifying the place of acidic foods. It only corrects errors and gives room for balance. An acidic individual or body increases the risk of infections from bacteria, yeast, parasites, and viruses. These microorganisms look for and grow efficiently in an acidic environment. To be candid, diseases that affect the vital organs of the body system like tooth decay, arthritis, heart diseases, etc., are most times linked to the level of acidity and alkalinity of the body.

Now, this is why taking a pH test is super important to your wellness and health. When a pH test is conducted, you become aware of whether your body is too acidic or too alkaline or in balance.

This is why a pH test is so important for your health. Testing your body pH will give you a sense of whether your body is tending toward metabolic acidity, or is in the balanced, slightly alkaline state that's necessary for healthy bones.

- STEPS TO TEST YOUR pH

1. First, get a pH test paper. This is readily available in chemists and pharmacist's shops. The pH paper is perfect for measuring the acid-alkaline level of any solution or aqueous substance. A low pH value, like we have discussed earlier, found at the end of the scale shows that you are in an acidic state while a high value of pH found on the higher end of the paper indicates an alkaline level.

2. The preferable time for this test is early in the morning this is because your first-morning urine and saliva (or before any meal at all and even before you brush your mouth) give the most accurate pH value and reading, though this isn't a compulsion.

- TO TEST WITH URINE:

    - Collect your urine in a little cup then dip the pH paper in the cup of urine entirely. Read the indication on the strip as you will be taught in a second.

- ## TO TEST USING SALIVA

  - First rinse your mouth very well like two to three times with water, spitting the water out at every time.

  - Then collect your saliva in a spoon (not cup this time, except you can give about 1 liter at that spot)

  - What you have to do next is to moisten the paper with that saliva from your spoon.

- 3. To read the result that comes as colors from the pH strip, there is always a chart at the back of your kit for the pH test strip, compare the color that your pH strip has now become with that. The color ranges from yellow to dark blue. Match your color to the particular color on the skit that corresponds to a number.

The pH value for normal urine is about 6.5 to about 7.5 while that of the saliva is between 7.0 to about 7.5

It is expedient to note that there could be a fluctuation in these values because of age differences. For an adult, it is still healthy to have a pH of 6.8 to 7.4, but there is an indication of a deficiency in the alkaline level. İt is beginning to turn acidic. For a young child, if the reading is between 7.0 to 7.5; this child is healthy.

You might ask, "what then do I do if my pH measures and reflects that I am acidic?"

Well, the good news is that you have nothing to fear. This state is reversible. You only need to take the right measures, and these right measures are explained simply and clearly in this book. Here is just a tip, keep in mind that you can consume 80% of alkaline-producing foods and 20% od acidic foods. Oh! You do not understand what I just said in that last line?! then you need to keep reading. This will be extensively discussed in this book. Keep reading!!!

CHAPTER 02

WHAT IS THE ALKALINE DIET?

Nowadays, it appears as though everyone, everywhere is talking about the 'Alkaline Diet.' It seems to have 'gained fame' recently. How famous!

"Oh! It's the alkaline diet that keeps me healthy," some keep reiterating. Others give credence to the alkaline diet for a job well done. Yet all things considered, what precisely is this food plan, and for what reason is it, how useful is the alkaline diet for the body? You wouldn't want to stop reading now, would you? Keep flipping! Treasures and mysteries yet to be found and unraveled.

The Alkaline Diet also referred to as the 'acid-alkaline balanced diet' or the 'antacid diet' is an eating routine remedy, though not strict, that emphasizes and suggests foods that balance the body's pH. The alkaline diet does this by the consuming more food that alkalizes the body, consequently increasing the pH, and wiping out food that promotes acidity. At the point when the body breaks down and uses food substances, a leftover is remaining toward the finish of the procedure. This leftover is referred to as ash. This ash is either acidic or alkaline, and subsequently influences the pH of organic liquids like urine and blood. The alkaline diet, therefore, is based on the principle that specific food influences the body's pH.

Caution: PLEASE counsel with your doctor before deploying any improvements to your eating regimen or prescriptions. This book is written just for informative purposes and isn't to be utilized for therapeutic guidance, conclusion or treatment.

In other words, the alkaline diet depends on the principle that what you eat influences the pH level, that is, the acidity or alkalinity, of your body. The eating regimen wipes out foods that have high acidic contents and emphasizes foods that are alkaline in nature.

HERE'S A LIST OF ALKALINE FOODS:

- Alkaline water

- Tofu

- Sprouts

- Goat or almond milk

- Herbal tea

- Gluten/yeast-free loaves of bread and wraps

- Sprouted pieces of bread and wraps

- Grasses including wheatgrass, grain, Kamut, shave and oat

- Nuts including coconut and almond

- Various seeds including flax, sunflower, sesame, and pumpkin

- Grains including amaranth, buckwheat, millet, quinoa and lentils

- Beans including pinto, red, soy, and white

- Vegetables including asparagus, broccoli, green beans, spinach, kale, sweet potatoes, eggplant, garlic, onion, celery, cucumber, lettuce, peas, pumpkin, squash and radishes

- Fruits including avocado, tomatoes, lemon, lime, grapefruit, new coconut, and pomegranate

- It is important to note that the alkaline diet encourages the consumption of food grown and cultivated from the soil. It tells you that it is essential to continue eating those foods that are planted and grown naturally. These foods are amazingly undiluted and provide natural minerals needed by the body.

In order to achieve balance, so many of the

foods you are accustomed to are what needs to be reduced.

Having an alkaline diet means eating 80% alkaline-producing foods and just 20% acid-producing ones. This might appear to be an overwhelming assignment; however, a better and comprehensive insight will be provided in the latter part of this book.

WHAT TO EAT

- Vegetables including verdant greens (spinach, lettuce, kale, cabbage) and carrots, green beans, cucumber, broccoli, artichokes, asparagus, peas, turnips, and that's just the beginning of the seeming 'difficult' task as most vegetables are alkaline-forming.

- Fruits like lemons and limes (they may appear to be strange, yet they are alkaline-producing), rhubarb, avocado, grapefruit, and tomato

- Beverages like almond milk, unsweetened soy milk, new vegetable juice, natural tea, vegetable soup, refined water, and lemon water (press a cut of lemon into your refined water)

- Nuts and grains, for example, almonds, pumpkin, and sunflower seeds spelled lentils, and any grown seeds

- Oils like olive, flaxseed, borage, avocado, and coconut

WHAT NOT TO EAT OR AT THE LEAST KEEP AWAY FROM

- Meats (What! Yes.., but if this is difficult, for a start, begin to substitute your meat with fish or just have a smaller portion)

- Dairy items

- Caffeinated refreshments, natural product juice, and liquor

- Fast foods, canned substances, microwaved dinners, etc.

- Yeast

- Sugar

- Chemically handled, produced or processed food.

The best method to help build a balanced pH is to eat parcel of supplement thick, alkalizing plant nourishments and to constrain your intake of fast foods/processed food. Since such huge numbers of various elements — gut wellbeing, stress, rest, drugs and therapeutic history — likewise influence how hard your body needs to function to keep up its suitable pH level, another way of life propensities can also be useful for re-establishing harmony.

80/20 RULE

WHAT IS THE 80/20 RULE?

This principle, 80/20 rule, that governs the alkaline diet suggests that you eat 80% alkaline foods, and 20% acidic nourishments. Note that:

- Every food that we eat gets to use, worked upon, and leaves behind ash, which is the reason once in a while, the alkaline diet is known as the alkaline ash diet. This leftover ash will either be alkaline- or acid-forming.

- When we are always giving the body nourishments that are acid-forming, it puts us at more severe danger of sickness and infection, for example, hypertension, cholesterol, coronary illness, and much disease. We are gradually making an acidic domain in the body.

- In the present moment, an acidic state can cause skin inflammation, low vitality, weight gain, torment, colitis, depression, and so on...

- In the long haul, an acidic body state can cause cerebrum issues, malignant growth, colitis, heart assault, stroke, obesity, and so forth...

10 TIPS FOR FOLLOWING THE 80/20 ALKALINE DIET:

You should know by now that how you live your life, including what you eat, has a significant role to play in your body pH balance. Below listed are ten tips on how to start, manage and create a pH balance in your body. Can you remember your nutritional worries? By the end of this list, they would be resolved. Trust me!

1. Reduce the quantity of an animal product in your meal. When you cut down on animal proteins, you do not just cut down on calories, but your circulatory and cholesterol strain is reduced to minimal. Consequently, the danger of coronary diseases, malignancy, and diabetes reduce drastically. Then the vegetables and entire grains that will replace the meat will help shield you from building up these incessant ailments, as well.

2. Start changing your eating routine continuously. After some time includes increasingly more alkaline-forming foods.

3. Be patient with yourself. Causing changes to how you to eat is basic, however difficult. Getting out from under negative behavior patterns and setting up new, solid schedules requires persistence. Understanding that occasionally disappointment is a piece of the procedure causes us to remain positive rather

than whipping ourselves

4. Drink a huge amount of water. According to Camelbak hydration master, Doug Casa, Ph.D., water makes up around 66% of our identity and impacts 100% of the procedures in our body. This explains why we feel better when we're drinking enough of it.

5. Persistence and consistency are cogent. Try to stay with the 80/20 rule as much as you can.

6. Get a lot of rest. Research has proven that you are bound to be more productive at your work and assignments when you get enough relaxation.

7. Eat appropriate, as your occupation demands. What a mason will consume as food shouldn't be what a pilot would neither will it be what a college boy will. Eat to suit you and your work type.

8. When you inhale profoundly, you increase the amount of the oxygen that is sent into your lungs, soothing pressure, and purifying your body from various collection of poisons. So breathe profoundly.

9. Chew your food properly. Did you know that it's been proven that as humans we can produce about two gallons of saliva a day?

10. Say no to junk food. As much as possible, avoid junk food. These junks are composed of

coloring, artificial sweeteners, preservatives, and other chemical substances that are highly unhealthy for the body. They are acid-forming too.

Keep in mind that this book isn't saying that all acid-forming foods are bad neither is it condemning the consumption of the foods. This book talks about creating balance, the right way through the right knowledge.

CHAPTER 03

ALKALINE SUPERFOOD LIST

As we have been discussing alkaline from chapter one, note that the food list given here doesn't suggest that there are no benefits of other types of food with a high concentration of acid not included here. Contrariwise, we are advocating that the alkaline concentrated food should be consumed more for optimum health. Likewise, every class of foods has its benefits, but you should consider taking conscious efforts in consuming alkaline foods than the acidic ones. Are you a vegan? Fine, you are not required to leave your eating habit. If you aren't a vegan, then you aren't required to be one. All that you have to do is to maintain the pattern of your food lifestyle but take into consideration that to maintain optimum health, consumption of alkaline foods is highly needful. In this chapter, we will look into a comprehensive list of alkaline superfoods. These foods are greatly rich in alkaline minerals and are recommended for eating. In addition to the listing, we would be learning the alkalinity level and other things relating to the foods listed.

VEGETABLES

- ARTICHOKES

This is a nice form of thistle fruit usually consumed when it is not mature. Generally, the alkaline level within the pH range is neutral mostly between 5.50 to 6.00. however, certain types of artichokes have their own range. The canned artichokes are usually between 4.30 to 4.60 because they are acidified. The french cooked artichokes are mostly in the range of 5.60 to 6.00. artichokes are cooked in Jerusalem are usually between the range of 5.93 to 6.00. By and large, a full artichoke has a moderate alkaline without any range of acidity, provided the preparation processes are not altered.

- ASPARAGUS (TIPS)

This type of vegetable is mostly consumed in spring. It is low in fat and calories. Additionally, it has both insoluble and soluble fiber, which is why most people prefer to take it as weight losing vegetable. The alkaline level is very high. Meanwhile, to get the fullest of the alkaline of Asparagus, one needs to consider the preparation processes, and the part consumed. For the buds of Asparagus, the range is usually 6.7. The cooked and canned ones are usually between 6.03 to 6.16 and 5.00 to 6.00, respectively. Asparagus could be frozen and cooked at the same time. When it undergoes these processes, the pH is always ranging from 6.35 to 6.48. the strained Asparagus would have between 4.80 to 5.09. lastly, asparagus that is green but canned when you consume them has between 5.20 to 5.32. Note that the preparations given here are to be examined carefully so that utmost efficiency would be attained in the joining of maintaining a healthy life.

- ## BAMBOO SHOOTS

Bamboo shoots could be canned, dried and fresh to be ready for consumption. They come in diverse shapes too. The bamboo shoots have between the range of 5.10 to 6.20 pH values. However, when you ====preseve the shoots, maybe by drying, the pH ranges between 3.50 to 4.60. They are very common in Asian dishes. Note that there are certain species of bamboo shoots mostly consumed. They include Phyllostachys, Bambusa vulgaris, etc.

- ## BROCCOLI

Broccoli is rich in vitamin C and K. The Alkaline level of broccoli is high. It aids digestion processes because it is a good source of fiber. The effect broccoli nutrients work amazingly in the body as it helps in areas such as keeping the bone strong, repairing tissues, etc. The pH level varies along with the preparation methods. Cooked broccoli will have between 6.30 to 6.52 while a frozen and cooked together will have 6.30 to 6.85. Additionally, canned broccoli will have approximately 5.20 to 6.80. So, you must consider these preparation means to be sure about the effect of alkalinity and acidity level.

• BEETROOTS

Beetroots, also called beet or red beet, are typically taproot of a beet plant, as the name implies. Upon consumption, they are good for control of dementia and blood pressure, maintenance of body stamina, and lots more. The alkalinity level is moderate. However, the pH level will be given based on the means of preparation. Without any alteration, beets will have approximately 5.30-6.60 level. Beets that are strained will have between the range of 5.32 to 5.56. A cooked beet will have 5.23 to 6.50, approximately. Although a canned and acidified beet will have between the range of 4.30 to 4.60, the only canned one will be between 4.90 and 5.80. Know the ones you have or will consume and maintain your balance using the standard scale given above.

• BRUSSELS SPROUTS

With edible and delicious buds, Brussels

sprouts are from the family of cabbages. The leaves are between the range of 1.5 cm to 4.0 cm in diameter long. This makes it very easy to add them to grains and they could be used as an accompaniment to many other foods. The alkalinity level is moderately alkaline. However, the pH level ranges from 6.00 to 6.30 approximately. Brussels sprouts are very rich in vitamins C, A, B6, and D. Additionally; They have cobalamin and calcium.

- CABBAGES

Cabbages are succulent leafy biennial plants. They come in different colors such as red, green, purple, etc. Based on their colors, they are classified into diverse varieties such as red cabbage, Chinese Cabbage, White Cabbage, etc. Meanwhile, all the varieties of cabbage have the same alkalinity level, which is moderately alkaline. To their pH levels, cabbage naturally its pH level ranging between 5.20 to 6.80. The red cabbage has its pH ranging from 5.60 to 6.00. The white cabbage has a pH level of around 6.2. Green cabbage has a pH level ranging from 5.50 to 6.75. Lastly, the savoy cabbage is mostly around 6.3.

- CARROTS

One thing about carrots is that they are neutrally concentrated in both alkaline and acid. In other words, they are mediating between acidity and alkalinity. The kind of calcium concentration in a cup of milk is equivalent to the one in just nine carrots. In their pH level, carrots generally have a level of 6. However, the preparation of carrots could influence the pH level they contain. A ground carrot will have between the range of 4.55 to 5.80. Canned carrots are mostly between the range of 5.18 to 5.22. Carrots that are strained mostly have a pH level ranging from 5.10 to 5.10. When carrots are cooked, they have another range of pH level, which is between 5.58 to 6.03. Lastly, when carrots are chopped, they have a pH level between 5.30 to 5.6.

- CELERY

Celery is mostly with an enlarged stalk that thrusts into larger leaves. They could be eaten raw or cooked. Among their health benefits is that they help to control blood pressure and heart diseases. In fact, they enhance the cognitive level irrespective of age. Amazingly, celery is highly concentrated in alkalinity. However, when celery is cooked, the pH level varies between 5.37 to 5.92. Though the pH level for celery without naturally ranges between 5.70 to 6.00, the knob of celery when is cooked has its level ranging between 5.71 to 5.85.

- DANDELIONS

Dandelions are flowering plants whose roots could be used in place of coffee. They are a good provider of antioxidants and maintaining the sugar level in the body. They have lots of health benefits contrary to what people believe about them as being wild plants. There are different types of dandelions, such as taraxacum, common dandelion, etc. The alkalinity level of dandelion green is high. They are good for healthy lifestyle maintenance, especially in adults.

• EGGPLANT

Eggplant is a common fruit with lots of names. It could be called aubergine and brinjal. Eggplant has a very low-calorie level, though the fiber is high. It is good for controlling weight, heart disease, and lots more. The alkaline level of eggplant is most times moderate. Note that the general pH level of an eggplant ranges between 5.50 to 6.50. Lastly, eggplant is rich in vitamins A, C, B-6, and D. Other nutrients in it include calcium, magnesium, iron, and cobalamin. It is delicious!

OTHER ALKALINE-FORMING VEGETABLES INCLUDE:

- Endives

- Garlic

- Green Beans

- Green Olives

- Dills

- Bell Peppers

- Cauliflowers

- Chard
- Chayote
- Chicory
- Chives
- Collard Greens
- Cucumbers
- Dulce
- Green Peas
- Greens (leafy)
- Kale
- Kelp
  - Leeks
- Lettuces
- Mustard Greens
- Okra
- Onions
- Oyster plants
- Parsley
- Parsnips
- Peas (fresh)
- Peppers

- Radishes

- Rutabagas

- Sea Veggies

- Spinach Sprouts (all)

- Summer squash

- Sweet Potatoes

- Swiss chard

- Tomatoes

- Turnips

- Watercress

- Wheat grass

- Wild Greens Dandelion Root

- Zucchini/Courgette

FRUITS

AVOCADOS

Avocados are very nice in the body system because they contain vitamins such as B, C and K. They are a good source of lots of nutrients to the body and fiber. The alkaline level of avocados is very high. You should dare to consume them thirty minutes before the main meal. Avocados have a pH level between the range of 6.27 to 6.58 generally. They have been proven to reduce the risk of heart-related diseases.

GRAPEFRUITS

Grapefruits are typically known for their large sour-sweet taste. They are citrus whose trees are mostly found in the subtropical region. The alkalinity level is commonly neutral. People always prefer grapefruits as a means of using them for weight loss. Grapefruit could have varying pH level, though. This is based on preparation methods. Grapefruits will have approximately 3.00 to 3.75. The canned grapefruits have between 3.08 to 3.32 while the ones that are canned and juiced simultaneously will range between 2.90 to 3.25.

TOMATOES

One of the most consumed fruits is tomatoes. Although many people believe they come from the southern part of America, they are found almost all over the continents. They are a good source of a flavor called umami. They could be eaten in diverse ways along which the pH level varies likewise. Typically, the alkalinity level of tomatoes is usually moderately alkaline. The pH level of tomatoes without any alteration in the preparation or that is fresh will be between 4.30 to 4.90, approximately. When tomatoes are used for soup with cream and canned, they could have 4.62 as their pH level. Tomato is used for wine when they are ripe and have a range of 4.42 to

4.56. Tomatoes are only canned will have a pH level between the range of 3.50 to 4.70. Tomatoes that are strained will have a range of 4.32 to 4.58, approximately. Tomato pastes will have a range of 3.50 to 4.70 as their pH level. Tomato juice should be between 4.10 to 4.60. Lastly, ground tomatoes have between the range of 4.30 to 4.47. Whichever way you want your tomatoes, you have been intimated on the pH level.

OTHER ALKALINE-FORMING FRUITS ARE:

- Lemons

- Limes

- Watermelon

- Oranges

- Banana

- Papaya

- Tangerines

- Strawberries

- Pineapples

- Raspberries

- Persimmon

OILS & FATS

AVOCADO OIL

Avocado oil is usually edible and good for cosmetics. It is used for cooking and lubrication. This oil is a means of preparing delicious dishes. It is a good source of fatty acids, vitamins, antioxidants, and lots more. The level of its alkalinity is usually neutral; in between acidity and alkalinity in their pH range.

COCONUT OIL

Coconut oil is mostly moderately alkaline concentrated. This type of oil doesn't get spoilt easily because it contains a low level of saturated fat. It has different types of applications. It is good for the skin too. It ensures sound health and mind all the time. Similarly, other alkaline-forming oils are:

- Flax Oil

- Hemp Seed Oil

- Olive Oil

- Sunflower Oil

- Sesame Oil

GRASSES & SPROUTS

- Alfalfa Alfalfa Sprouts

- Amaranth Sprouts

- Barley Grass

- Broccoli Sprouts

- Dog Grass

- Fenugreek Sprouts

- Kamut Grass

- Kamut Sprouts

- Lemon Grass

- Millet Sprouts

- Mung Bean Sprouts

- Oat Grass

- Quinoa Sprouts

- Shave Grass

- Spelt Sprouts

- Wheat Grass

GRAINS, CEREALS & BREAD

BUCKWHEAT

Often mistaken for a grain, buckwheat is edible. It is not a grain, but it could be processed to flour or eaten as a whole. The alkalinity concentration of a whole and flour buckwheat is mostly moderate.

Whatever the processing methods used on buckwheat before consumption, they maintain not-too-acidic-and-not-too-alkaline in the body. To say, buckwheat tries to strike a balance to maintain a good pH level. One of the richest nutrients in buckwheat is protein. Other things contained in it include antioxidant, magnesium, fiber, few specified proteins, and copper. If your goal is to lose weight, buckwheat should be your friend from now on. Others are:

- Kamut

- Millet

- Amaranth

- Quinoa

- Spelt

- Sprouted Bread

- Sprouted Tortillas

- Yeast-Free Bread

- Dehydrated flax seed crackers

NUTS & SEEDS

- Almond Butter

- Almonds

- Carraway Seeds

- Cumin Seeds
- Fennel Seeds
- Hemp Seeds
- Pumpkin Seeds
- Sesame Seeds
- Sunflower Seeds

DRINKS

- Alkaline Water
- Barley Grass Juice
- Coconut Water
- Fresh Lemon &
- Lime Water

FRESH VEGETABLE JUICES

- Green Drinks
- Green Tea
- Herbal Tea
- Wheat Grass

CONDIMENTS & SPICES

- Unfermented Soy)

- Almond Butter

- Bee Pollen

- Bragg Aminos

- Chili Pepper

- Cinnamon

- Curry Powders

- Ginger Guacamole (fresh made)

HERBS (ALL)

WHY IS IT GOOD TO DRINK ALKALINE WATER?

Alkaline water is known for the following properties

1. It supports the immune system

2. It helps get rid of mineral deficiencies

3. It stabilizes the body's pH and nullifies dehydration

4. It has certain anti-aging properties

5. It aids mental clarity and enhances focus

6. It improves energy, endurance, and stamina.

7. In fact, it is six times more hydrating than the average 'pure' water.

8. From various studies, it has been noted that

the intake of alkaline water reduces platelet aggregation and improves blood flow.

9. Finally, an acidic environment, that should have support health problems like inflammation, cancer, infections, diabetes, etc., is not permitted.

10. It would please you to know that alkaline water helps with

1. Fatigue

2. Heartburn

3. Digestive issues

4. Cramps

5. High blood pressure

6. Diarrhea

7. Regulating blood sugar.

8. Joint pains

9. Constipation

10. Migraines

11. Nausea

12. Stress

13. Weight issues and the list goes on.

It is notable to know that alkaline water acts as an anti-oxidant. Anti-oxidants are substances that act to prevent or slow down the oxidation of other chemicals. It is a group of vitamins that acts against the effects of other things such as free radicals. Free radicals, on the other hand, is a molecule that is highly reactive and unpredictive. Antioxidants can help prevent diseases like cancer, cardiovascular disease, immune dysfunction, and much more. They are essential to be present in almost all the classes of food consumed within 24hrs; this will help you strike lots of balances in chemical breakdown processes in the body.

Oxidation-Reduction Potential, called by the acronym ORP is a way of measuring the amount of antioxidant by testing its electrical charge (that is, '+' or '-')

A positive ORP interprets that a lot of free radicals are present in that water while a negative ORP contains quite an amount of antioxidants.

In summary, Positive ORP = free radicals (which is EXTREMELY BAD)

Negative ORP = Antioxidants (this water is good)

Alkaline ionized water has a strong negative ORP and contains a lot of electrons that will be readily donated to unusual or not perfectly circular oxygen radicals in order to block the interaction of this active oxygen with normal molecules.

CHAPTER 04

HOW DOES ACIDIC FOOD AFFECT THE BODY?

Have you been questing how that it is possible to know if a food is acidic or alkaline? Would you love to be able to tell, just be the look while shopping and moving across the grocery store or restaurants, that food is either acidic or alkaline?

There are two basic methods otherwise called tests that can be used to know whether a food is acidic or alkaline and a primary difference between these methods. This classification is what most alkaline food charts are based on. The key difference between these methods determines whether its usage is correct or not. This explains the inconsistencies between the lists and classifications.

THESE METHODS ARE

- PRAL method

- The effect on the body

PRAL METHOD.

PRAL stands for 'Potential Renal Acid Load.' It is a method used to accurately check for the acidity of food by burning it down to a residue referred to as ash and then the pH of the ash is checked. It is accurate for a vast number of uses but can be practically misleading for an alkaline diet.

This method burns away the sugar and yeast present in the food, whereas these two are important determinants to ascertain whether a food is alkaline-forming or acid-forming.

What the important key is that in checking a food. It isn't to check whether a food is acidic or alkaline. But to check whether the food is acid-forming or alkaline-forming to the body that consumes such.

When you understand this key, you are already on your way to a piece of great knowledge. This explains why most charts have all fruits as alkaline-forming because the PRAL method has already burnt off all the sugar that should have indicated that is it acid-forming.

"THE EFFECT ON THE BODY" METHOD.

This method is based on the research work of Dr. Robert Young, who is a major researcher of the alkaline diet. He, over time, he has gathered a list of foods and has grouped them as either acid-forming or alkaline-forming by checking through analysis of his blood samples over 150,000 live blood analysis tests. This approach has produced results and can be followed as trustworthy. It is simple but effective. Just give it a try.

Generally speaking, there are two types of foods, and they are basically:

- Fresh foods

- Packaged ones

With the aid of simple thoughts and common sense, you have all the clues to apply this test. These clues aren't misleading. To check if a food is alkaline-forming, note the following:

- IS THE FOOD FRESH?

Most fresh foods are alkaline-forming. They are always more alkaline-forming because they still have their nutrients intact and have not been processed or made acidic through the process.

- WHAT IS THE FOOD'S MINERAL CONTENT?

Predominantly, alkaline foods contain a lot of alkaline minerals. These alkaline minerals include calcium, sodium bicarbonate, manganese, iron, potassium, and magnesium.

- WHAT IS THE FOOD'S SUGAR CONTENT?

All sugars, whether fructose, galactose, glucose, etc., are extremely acid-forming in the body. Certain fruits contain a very high level of fructose and are therefore acid-forming.

- IS IT A VEGGIE?

Almost all, if not all vegetables are between slightly alkaline-forming to highly alkaline-forming. Therefore, they are on the list of alkaline foods.

- WHAT IS ITS COLOR?

Once it is green, it is an indication that it contains the green pigment- chlorophyll. Chlorophyll is a very alkaline-forming substance.

- WHAT IS ITS WATER CONTENT?

High water content equals high alkaline-forming, while low water level may be an indication that the food is acid-forming.

In addition to the above-stated clues, other factors that be used to check if a food is acid-forming are:

- DOES THE FOOD CONTAIN YEAST?

Foods containing yeast are high acid-forming foods too. They are on the 'No list' also when you are in for the alkaline diet.

- FERMENTED OR NOT?

Fermented foods are highly acid-forming. The

fermentation process makes food acidic.

- IS IT REFINED OR PROCESSED?

The fresh food is always the best. The more cooked/processed or refined a food is, the more acidic it probably will be.

Now, Even without your food chart, you should by yourself be able to select foods that are alkaline-forming and stay off acid-forming foods just by seeing it.

An average American diet contains a high amount of calories, fat, sugars and not enough vegetables, fibers, whole grain, etc. However, the place of balance cannot be overemphasized. It is crucial to keeping the mind and body in good health. A well-balanced array of food provides essential vitamins and minerals. It prevents diseases, because a balanced body and appropriate amounts of required nutrient (carbohydrate, fats, protein, fiber...) give the body strength, improve the brain's function and keep the body at a healthy weight. An unhealthy diet is very risky, as many diseases in our world today are a result of this unhealthy/unbalanced diets.

WHY IS IT BAD TO CONSUME TOO MANY ACID-FORMING FOODS?

A diet that contains too many acid-forming foods can make the urine acidic, which leads to other negative health effects like the formation of uric acid stones in the kidney. It has also been suggested that too much acid-forming food can cause deterioration in the bones and muscle. When the body is becoming too acidic, calcium, which is contained in the bones, is adopted and used to restore the body's pH. This leads to a deterioration in the bones and muscle. Let us not forget that too much acidic opens the gateway for other diseases such as cancer, heart and liver diseases, etc.

I, therefore, humbly advice that you limit your consumption of acid-forming foods and resort to acid-base balanced diets. All of the wrong food choices have been affecting your health negatively over the years.

From Clemson University, we can deduce a list of foods from most acidic (yet alkaline-forming) to the least:

- FOOD PH VALUE

1. Lemon juice 2.00- 2.60

2. Limes 2.00- 2.80

3. Blue plums 2.80- 3.82

4. Grapes 2.90-3.82

5. Pomegranates 2.93-3,20

6. Grapefruits 3.00-3.75

7. Blueberries 3.12-3.33

8. Pineapples 3.20-4.00

9. Apples 3.30-4.05

10. Peaches 3.30-4.05

11. Oranges 3.69-4.34

12. Tomatoes 4.30-4.90

HERE IS A LIST OF VEGETABLES AND THEIR RESPECTIVE PH LEVELS:

VEGETABLE PH VALUE

1. Sauerkraut 3.30-3.60

2. Cabbage 5.20-6.80

3. 3. Beets 5.30-6.60

4. Corn 5.90-7.50

5. Mushrooms 6.00-6.70

6. Brocolli 6.30-6.85

7. Collard green 6.50-7.50

CHAPTER 05

WHY THE WESTERN DIET KEEPS MAKING US SICK?

Did you know that following the Western diet increases your risk of chronic illness and early death?

Changing the way you eat is capable of helping you live healthier and longer.

The typical processed western foods such as hamburger, pizza, grilled chicken and chips, hot dogs, etc., are tied to so many health problems. It increases the risk of chronic diseases and can eventually lead to an early death.

According to statistic and the 2015-2020 dietary guidelines for Americans report, more than a third of a quarter of adults and one- third of little children and youths in America are overweight and obese.

Over the years, in addition to the effect of unhealthy, imbalance and processed foods, little or no exercise and enough sleep have been contributing factors to the incidence of chronic diseases in the western world.

It is saddening to know that about half of Americans have at least one diet-related chronic diseases: Heart disease, obesity, high blood pressure, diabetes, some cancer types, and the list goes on.

You might want to ask. What exactly are these western diets? Why do people even eat them?

The western food is made up of food that is composed of refined sugars, saturated fats, little fiber, and also little to no healthy fats. So, from this definition, most processed foods fall into this category. Ultra-processed foods contain a high amount of sodium, synthetic trans fats, flavors, and artificial sweeteners. All of these are added to the products to increase their shelf storage and preservation time.

SOME OF THESE WESTERN/ PROCESSED FOODS INCLUDE:

- Potato chips

- Bread (particularly, white bread)

- Cakes

- Packaged Snack

- Pizza

- Candy

- Soft drinks

BUT WHY DO PEOPLE EAT THEM?

Processed foods are super appealing, convenient, and tasty. We at times are too busy with life's works and problems, so we end up assuming there is no time to cook. So, we settle for what is available, which in most cases is fast food, and these foods are very cheap.

The conventional and western diet may be cheap now, but it will get costly when it makes you sick and reduces the quality of your life because of your body's lack of energy. In the digestive system, certain microorganisms that are collectively named microbiome help the body to digest food, regulate metabolism, prevent infections, and control the immune system. Now, research has shown that when a diet high in fat and sugar (acid-forming food) is ingested, it kills the essential bacteria in the gut and this leads to an imbalance in the body's mechanism which could further lead to malfunctions.

Typically, certain types of bacteria are present in the gut, and these bacteria depend on a healthy yet diverse diet, but with the recent chronic consumption of Western diet, many of these bacteria have disappeared. These microbiome present in the gut are essential for healthy living. Therefore, when not present or compromised, diseases are the result. From this, we get to know that the western diet is not ideal and can be catastrophic.

The result of the Western diet on the immune system is that the body is kept in chronic, low-grade inflammation. At this state, the immune system sees and acknowledge some stimuli as an infection or threat. This might be right for a few stimuli, but others may not be threats at all, this then makes the immune system of the body attack itself (Its own cells, tissues, and organs.) This phenomenon is called Autoimmunity.

Therefore, changing your diet may be one way to reduce these problems of Autoimmunity or and chronic inflammation. Because it is assumed that what you eat is what dictates the phenomenon your body undergoes.

According to the 2015-2020 Dietary Guidelines for Americans: One-fourth of the American population are not eating healthy meals, vegetable, and fruits, although research has proven that the health of adults, who have chronic health conditions improves and gets better progressively when they start to eat healthier and live actively. There is an urgent call to improve our meals and eating habits. It might not be so easy, but we have to make better food choices. You must understand that to live healthily; you need to live a healthier lifestyle.

HERE IS WHAT YOU CAN START DOING TODAY TO IMPROVE YOUR HEALTH:

- EAT LESS SALT AND SUGAR.

According to the CDC, though about one teaspoon of salt is recommended for daily consumption, 9 out of 10 Americans consume more. In the same vein, sugar should be consumed at the rate of not more than six teaspoons per day for women and nine teaspoons per day for men, but the average American consumes about 19.5 teaspoons every day. Can you see how endangered we are? Hence, to live a healthy life and have more energy, we should eat less salt and sugar.

- CONSUME MORE PLANT-BASED FOODS

In the course of this study, we have mentioned several times that instead of refined grains and processed/synthetic foods, we are advised to choose more vegetables, fruits, herbs, spices, legumes, and high fiber-containing foods.

- REPLACE BAD FAT WITH THE HEALTHY FAT.

Fats found in foods like the salmon and oils from plants such as olive, canola, some nuts, and seeds are mostly healthy when eaten moderately. You should replace unhealthy fats and oils with these healthy ones.

- NOT ALL PROCESSED FOODS ARE UNHEALTHY. CHOOSE ACCURATELY.

Certain foods have been processed minimally and still contain a good amount of nutrients. In fact, whole foods like fruits and fresh vegetables had gone through specific processes before they made it to the shelves. In order to aid your search for processed foods that are still healthy, we have provided a list below.

- Canned beans

- Frozen fruits and vegetables

- Whole-grain pasta

- Nut butter and packaged nuts

- Dairy-free milk and yogurt

- Hummus

- Canned and frozen fish

Though the developing world is advancing towards urbanization and there is a progressive shift to the urban lifestyle which implies less activity and more consumption of the western diet, we must consider bad eating habits and unhealthy foods to be same as smoking cigarettes. Teach young kids about healthy eating habits from a very early age. And just like we do not want people to smoke or even do that around our kids, we should behave in like manner towards unhealthy food.

WHAT IS THE WESTERN DIET?

FEATURES OF THE WESTERN DIET INCLUDES

- Over-consumption of over-refined sugars

- Consumption of saturated fats

- High consumption of animal proteins

- A reduced intake of plants, vegetables, and plant-based fibers.

- This, consequently, translates to a diet that is

- High in Salts

- Sugar

- Red meat

- Fats

- And low fiber content

- In summary, this results in

- Too many calories.

- Increased risk of infection

Western meals that are characterized by highly refined/processed foods throw off the immune system of the body. Causing adverse effects on health and optimum balance.

Foods that contain fructose and palmitic acid (as found in candy bars) are agents that cause a shift in the normal functioning of the body, especially the function of the immune system.

Most times, the body confuses a particular nutrient in excess like the palmitic acid for a bacteria. Then, the body starts to fight the palmitic acid, supposing it to be a bacteria; this is not healthy! It results in terrible health conditions like Autoimmunity. When the real infection sets in, the immune system is distracted and unable to face the real danger, the body is thrown off, and the situation gets worsened. However, this effect is not permanent, and it can be reversed.

The solution to this effect will be a change in diet. Once your body is exposed to a different and a change in diet (that is, the Acid-Alkaline Diet), it will remove the toxins, and excess acids will be removed from the body. The perfect immune activity then gets restored and starts to function normally again.

OBESITY AND DIABETES

Obesity It makes the body susceptible to other diseases. The rate at which obesity is recorded globally has increased over the years due to a simultaneous increase of unhealthy food consumption, especially junk foods that are extremely rich in calories and fats. According to statistics from the WHO (World Health Organization), in 2014, adults that were obese were over six hundred million. In that same year, about two billion adults were seen as overweight.

Obesity is very unhealthy. It serves a gate for

other diseases and infections. In obese people, inflammation rate is very high, and this is why there is an increased rate of heart diseases, arthritis, cancer, and stroke in them.

Most joints conditions and inflammations, like gout and arthritis, are ascribed to obesity, the increase in obesity level is also a contributing factor to the rise in cases of joint, hip, and knee replacement. This is due to the extra pressure that is placed on the joint.

In the same vein and linked to obesity is diabetes. It was said to have affected about 374 million people in 2014, isn't this disheartening?

According to the IDF diabetes atlas, the development of Type II diabetes is linked with diet and numbers are rising in every country. So many countries have recorded death in several regions as a result of this diabetes. It is a pity that it can be hereditary too.

CANCER RISK

The western diet has been linked to an increased risk of cancer, particularly colon and prostate concern in men. From observation, men who consume Western diets at a regular frequency have been found to have 2.5 times the risk of prostate cancer.

Colon cancer is linked to the inflammation

caused by a change in the activities of the gut bacteria. Americans, due to their diet routines and junk foods, have about 50 times more risk rate of having colon cancer. This is problematic because it, over time, reduces the genetic variation and consequently, results in disease development. Inflammation in the colon can damage cells and cause an increased form of cell death in the affected area.

It is now clearly seen that diet plays an essential role in the health of the world's population. This is why there is an urgent need to call the awareness of people to fix their diets. This is the primary call of this book. I hope you are learning.

CHAPTER 06

ALKALIZING HERBS AND SUPPLEMENTS

Do you want a healthy body? Of course, yes. From our daily activities to the kinds of food we eat, our utmost desire is to maintain a healthy living. The beginning of healthy life could be attributed to alkalizing your body; this is quite simple. Although on the spectrum, acid and alkaline are sides of two opposite things, alkaline is quite useful to the body than acid. In the real sense, the body supposed to be alkaline, but in most people, it is not. This is because many of us are stressed out too often, consume sugar at a high rate, and consume meat at a high level. For a healthy state of mind and life, you must maintain the balance of the pH level in the body. The excessive acidity of the body is quite detrimental to it. Based on the fact that most people's body has a high rate of acidity, one of the cures is to use supplements. These are not to be confused or seen as a balanced diet, but instead they help the body to be more alkaline. Before you use any supplements, try to consult professionals. This will save you from side effects and future risk you might be exposed to. There is now the need to maintain a good pH level. Seeing that pH level is a combination of acidity and alkaline concentration. The following are different ways to increase and maintain good body acid-alkaline balance naturally:

ALWAYS EAT AN ALKALINE DIET

Knowing fully well your aim (maintaining alkaline body), you must always be willing and ready to consume lots of alkaline food. Food items such as wild rice, green tea, fruits, vegetables, etc. are samples you should consume.

On the other hand, you could try to reduce the acidity rate by simply reducing sugar, dairy, meat, alcohol, etc. Without any form of formal treatment, you will notice changes in your health status and body metabolism. Note that by consuming alkaline related food directly, scientists have little reservation of how it could affect your health. Nevertheless, advantages such as weight loss, inflammation control, increase in immunity, and increase in lifespan are possible with the alkaline diet.

Early in the morning, try to engage in Yoga exercises and meditation for a considerably long period of time. This activity will significantly reduce your stress levels, which will result in a reduction of acidity rate in the body automatically.

EMBRACE TURMERIC AND COCONUT OIL

Turmeric is an herb with great importance on health maintenance. Make turmeric your friend. Coconut oil also has many health benefits. You could either add to your food or even use it to fry. It is very good for your body. You can incorporate these tow superfoods into your vegetables too, and they will be of immense help.

BODY MASSAGE

It is a fact that body massage could help in the removal of toxins in the body. There is an increase in mental and nervous system health status with good body massage. To ensure a good alkaline body, always try to do body massage by yourself or any other persons. This will help you a lot. To do this, simply put coconut oil round all your body parts, then massage gently

REDUCTION IN COFFEE INTAKE

For a good alkaline body, try to alternate your morning coffee intake. It could be a bit difficult, but nothing is more important than being healthy. To maintain a good alkaline body, always a reduction in coffee intake.

The following are types of supplements that can be used in the alkalizing of your body;

ALKALIZING THROUGH CALCIUM SUPPLEMENTS

In a bid to cope with the removal of acidity in the body, oftentimes, the body loses more calcium, which makes it detrimental to the health. In order to maintain balance and restore calcium, you must be willing to take minerals always as supplements.

ALKALIZING THROUGH THE POWDER OF GREEN FOOD

There are various types of green powder that could be used to alkalize your body. These are made from chlorella algae and some juice types such as alfalfa, barley, and wheat. Although many people take these powders as an ingredient of water that is a swamp, adding them to your smoothies, water, etc. will work wonders in your body system. In fact, they help your body to in the promotion of energy, fight against illness, improved energy, and less body pain. There are amazing powders.

ALKALIZING THROUGH PH DROPS OR POWDER

In the formulation of the market, there are some things specifically designed to enhance health and body mechanism. These usually contain a solution of chlorine dioxide or hydrogen peroxide which releases oxygen in your body. More so, they help to restore biochemical balance in the body. They are mostly called pH drops or powder, though there are other names for them too. Minerals and salt such as potassium, magnesium, manganese, calcium, and iron are contained in these powders most times.

DISCLAIMER:

Many of the following herbs have poisonous and dangerous effects if used incorrectly, especially in cases such as pregnancy and breast-feeding.

The following list gives you a very general overview and is written for educational purposes only, not a substitute for the medical advice of a trained health professional. If you decide to use any of these herbs, please do so under medical supervision.

All herbs, especially the bitter ones, are considered as alkalizing by the herb specialists.

The following herbs have healing and reversing disease soothes. Herbs that are highly rich in alkaline include;

1. **ARNICA**

Origin: North America

USAGE: Arnica is used as a cream. Arnica is an anti-inflammatory and antiseptic herb. It is an effective and powerful treatment for external wounds. It promotes tissue regeneration and relieves pains. It treats arthritis, sprains, bruises, and headaches.

PRECAUTION: it is for external use only. It is toxic when ingested. Pregnant or breast-feeding woman should stay away from arnica.

1. **BATANA OIL**

Origin: Honduras, Central, and South America

USAGE: Batana Oil is made from the fruit of the Elaeis oleifera tree. The oil is rich in fatty acids, nutrients, and phytonutrients. It helps strengthen the hair, promoting its growth and restoring it to its original color.

PRECAUTION: it is for external use only.

1. **BLADDERWRACK**

Origin: Atlantic Ocean, Pacific Ocean, North Sea,

Baltic Sea.

USAGE: Bladderwrack is a rich source of iodine. It is also rich in magnesium, potassium, and calcium. Bladderwrack is a great way to help and cure iodine deficiency. Bladderwrack is proven to have an amazing effect of reducing anti-estrogenic effects. It lowers the risk of estrogen-dependent diseases. This means the herb is super-efficient in ladies since estrogen is the female hormone. Bladderwrack lowers cholesterol and lipid level and hence a great aid with weight loss.

PRECAUTION: It is not safe to take bladderwrack by mouth; it is for external use only. Pregnant or breast-feeding woman should stay away from this herb.

2. BLESSED THISTLE

Origin: Mediterranean

USAGE: blessed thistle is rich in iron and has been used for traditional medicine. It helps increase oxygen flow and circulation to the brain, to help it function well alongside the lungs and heart. It is bitter but works wonders on the liver and gallbladder. It has been employed and used to remove toxins from the body even to intracellular cleansing.

PRECAUTION: Be sure to consult your doctor before use in cases of allergies. Pregnant women and lactating mothers are warned to seek medical advice before use, too.

3. CASCARA SAGRADA

Origin: Western North America

USAGE: Cascara Sagrada is a laxative. It contains Emodin which has anticancer and antiviral properties. It also initiates the peristaltic movement of the intestine, moving dates and toxins through the intestine till it is gotten rid of. It is a healthy herb for the liver, stomach, intestine, and pancreas.

PRECAUTION: if you have or do develop abdominal pain, this herb is not advised. Pregnant women are, likewise, not advised to use it as it can induce labor. Lactating mothers can pass this too to there children while breastfeeding.

4. CONTRIBO

Origin: South America

USAGE: Contribo is used in traditional medicine for arthritis and edema, to stimulate the immune system and white blood cell production, to kill parasites, and to treat snakebites. This herb can be very dangerous if not used correctly. Precautions: Women who are pregnant or nursing should avoid contribo.

5. CHAPARRAL

Origin: Mexico, Southwest North America

USAGE: chaparral has antimicrobial and

antibacterial, antitumor and anticancer, and antiulcerogenic and anti-inflammatory properties, all in one. Chaparral improves skin health by treating skin conditions like rashes, bruises, psoriasis, and eczema. It has an antiparasitic effect too, hence its use in addressing sexually transmitted diseases by killing the parasites responsible. Finally, it is used as an expectorant to treat respiratory problems like bronchitis and cold.

PRECAUTIONS: When Chaparral is taken in a dose higher than recommended, it could cause liver damage.

6. DAMIANA

Origin: Mexico, Central, and South America and the Caribbean.

USAGE: Damiana is used by both men and women to strengthen the sexual organs and boost sexual drive and potency. Damiana is known for balance because it helps in balancing the testosterone and estrogen level in men and women, respectively. It is used to treat constipation because it also stimulates the churning out the intestinal tract.

7. COCOLMECA

Origin: Mexico, Jamaica

USAGE: Cocolmeca is a kind of plant that is from the Smilax genus. It works as an anticancer, antioxidant, anti-inflammatory, and antiulcer herb having diuretic properties. Cocolmeca works by binding with toxins and expelling them from the body.

8. ELDERBERRY

Origin: America, Africa, Asia, Europe

Elderberry has properties that act against inflammations, viral infection, cancer, and influenza. Therefore, it is a remedy for cold, flu, and allergies.it is also used to remove mucus from the respiratory system.

PRECAUTIONS: Elderberry comes in different species, and most of these are toxic. Sambucus nigra, a species, is known to be non-toxic and has been used for medical purposes.

9. EYEBRIGHT

The origin of Eyebright is unknown.

Eyebright has anti-inflammatory and antiseptic properties and is used to as an eyewash to treat all forms of inflammation of the eyes, particularly the chronic ones. İt also has some soothing effect that works on the mucous membrane of the eye. Eyebright is used to treat wounds on the skin too. For the eyes, it works to treat blepharitis bacterial infection and conjunctivitis.

10. GUACO

Origin: South America, Jamaica

USAGE: Guaco has certain healthy properties

such a the anti-inflammatory, antiallergic, and bronchodilator. Primarily, in traditional medicine, Guaco is used for upper respiratory problems like asthma, colds, bronchitis, and flu. As an anti-inflammatory effect, guaco works for the inflammation of the digestive tract and rheumatoid arthritis. As an anti-bacterial effect, it cures yeast infection and candida.

11. HUEREQUE

Origin: Central and South America, Jamaica, and the Caribbean.

USAGE: Huereque is known as an antiobesity, hypoglycemic, and antimicrobial medicinal herb. İt is used to lower blood sugar levels. İt can also treat diabetes and help you reduce weight. It has a cleansing effect on the pancreas.

12. HOMBRE GRANDE

Origin: The Caribbean, Jamaica, Central, and South America

USAGE: Hombre Grande can be used as an insecticide, and against fungal infections, malaria, ulcer, and cancer. İts primary use in traditional medicine is to treat measles on the skin and constipation/diarrhea and fever, via oral administration. İt also stimulates the digestive tract and the production of bile. İt has been used to improve and increase appetite and to cleanse the blood. To support and enhance the immune system, Hombre grande functions in re-balancing the digestive tract microflora.

13. HOPS

Origin: Germany

Hops, just like most of the medicinal plants (herbs), has anticancer, antibacterial, and anti-inflammatory properties.

Hops help relieve pains, enhance urination and appetite, promote digestion, fight insomnia, reduce tension, anxiety, and nervousness, to mention but a few.

14. HYDRANGEA

Origin: Northeastern Asia, Southwestern United States

Hydrangea Root has anti-inflammatory, lithotrophic, antiseptic, antiparasitic, and autoimmune properties. Hydrangea dissolves calcium deposits in soft tissues, and this effect is due to the presence of a compound named Hydrangin in the Hydrangea herb. İt can and has been used to treat bladder and kidney disease like dissolving kidney stones and cleaning the lymphatic system.

15. LAVENDER

Origin: Africa, Canary Islands, Mediterranean, Asia, India

Lavender has many positive effects on health. It is known to be

- An antifungal medicinal herb

- Antibacterial medicinal herb

- Analgesic medicinal herb medicinal herb

- Anti-inflammatory medicinal herb

- Anti-insomnia Medicinal herb

- Anticonvulsant Medicinal herb

- Antispasmodic Medicinal herb

- Antianxiety Medicinal herb

- Antidepressant medicinal herb

WOW! WHAT A LIST!

In traditional medicine, Lavender is used in treating abdominal swelling resulting from gas, depression, stomach upset, migraine, nausea, joint pains, vomiting, restlessness, nerve pains, loss of appetite and insomnia.

16. LILY OF THE VALLEY

Origin: Europe, Northern Asia

Lily of the Valley has been used for several years now by several people, especially by the herb specialists. It has the following properties: Diuretic, antitumor, and anti-angiogenic. Lily of the valley is used to treat heart failure and heartbeats that are irregular. It treats dropsy and debility. All of these are possible because Lily of the valley increases oxygen transportation to the heart, thereby, reducing blood pressure.

PRECAUTIONS: it is not recommended for pregnant women. It is advised that the lily of the valley shouldn't be taken without provision supervision.

17. NETTLE

Origin: North Africa, Asia, Western North America

Nettle has antiulcer, analgesic, anti-inflammatory, diuretic, anticancer, antioxidant, and antimicrobial properties. The root of the nettle root is used for joints, as an enlarged prostate, and for diuretic purposes. The leaves are for hair loss, anemia, arthritis, eczema, sore muscles, rash, diabetes, enlarged spleen, and asthma. Nettle cleanses the blood and works as a great and healthy health tonic.

18. NOPAL

Origin: Mexico, Central America, the Caribbean, Western

United States, Eastern United States

Nopal has many phytochemicals, minerals, antioxidants, and vitamins. It can be used to treat type II diabetes, obesity, colitis, diarrhea, viral infections, and alcohol handover.

19. PRODIGIOSA

Origin: Southwestern North America, New Mexico

To stimulate the pancreas and the liver secretion, Prodigiosa is used. It is known for cleansing of the bile, liver, and gallbladder. It can treat headaches, fever, stomach pain, diarrhea, diabetes, and diseases of the gallbladder.

20. RED CLOVER

Origin: Northwest Africa, Western Asia.

Red clover herb has been proven to have anti-cancer, diuretic, expectorant, and sedative, anti-inflammatory, and antiatherosclerosis properties. It works to relieve symptoms from menopause because of its estrogen properties. It also works perfectly to break calcium build up in soft tissues, purifying the blood, and cleaning away fluid wastes from the lymphatic system.

21. RHUBARB ROOT

Origin: China

Rhubarb root has antioxidant, heavy-metal chelation, anticancer, and antibacterial properties. Rhubarb root treats digestive system issues like diarrhea, constipation, acid reflux, and stomach pain by regulating the tract. This herb softens stool in order to ease the bowel movements and prevent it from tearing the anus lining. To treat kidney stones, Rhubarb root is a great pick.

22. SAGE

Origin: Mediterranean

Low-density lipoproteins and cholesterol are

the unhealthy kinds of cholesterol and lipids in the body. While high-density lipoproteins are the healthy ones. Sage is said to reduce the level of the bad lipids and increase/improve the good lipids, thereby balancing the ratio. Sage is an anti-inflammatory, antitumor, antioxidant, and antiobesity herb. İt improves memory, treat diabetes, nourish the pancreas, and reduce gastrointestinal inflammation.

23. SANTA MARIA

Origin: Central America, Mexico

The attributes of Santa Maria include Antidepressant, antifungal, antioxidant, analgesic, and antibacterial effects. It can be used to treat abdominal pains, diarrhea, rheumatism, respiratory diseases, and skin issues. It has been used by Psychiatrists to relax the nerves.

24. SAPO

Origin: Central America, Mexico

Gall stones and kidney treatments seem to be a unique train to most alkaline herbs. Sapo is not excluded has it also works to treat those. İt is an antioxidant having anti-inflammatory properties. İt lowers triacylglycerol and cholesterol level in the arteries and blood.

25. SARSAPARILLA

Origin: Mexico, Jamaica, India, South America.

This herb is in two species.

Smilax that comes from South America

Hemidesmus indicus that finds its origin from India.

These two are similar in look and properties. They have medicinal properties like the anticancer, antiulcer, anti-inflammatory, and diuretic.

Sarsaparilla helps detoxify the blood and body by binding to the toxins to expel them from the system. İn traditional, it treats skin conditions like leprosy, pains like headache, joint pain, and sexual impotences too.

26. SEA MOSS

Origin: Atlantic Ocean coastal area

Sea moss has antibacterial, anti-inflammatory, and laxative properties. Sea moss is to soothe irritated mucous membranes from colds, coughs, bronchitis, tuberculosis, gastric ulcers, and intestinal problems. Sea moss is used to support skin and joint health, and its wide range of nutrients serve as a natural mineral supplement.

27. SENSITIVA

Origin: Central America

USAGE: Sensitiva like the word "sensitive" is known to increase sexual sensitivity(desire). It is an antidepressant, antibacterial, anti-inflammatory, and antioxidant herb. It treats uterine infections, stops bleeding, and stops arthritis pain and hemorrhoid.

28. SHEA BUTTER

Origin: Shea Butter finds its origin from Africa.

The Shea butter is got from the Shea tree nut. It is a traditional plant. It is famous for its ability on the skin to provide protective nutrients such as the fatty acid and shields the skin from UV light. İt moisturizes the skin, treats blemishes, eczema, sunburn, and wounds. İt also increases the elasticity of the skin.

29. TILA/BASSWOOD/LINDEN

Origin: North America, Asia, Europe

Tila is used to

Support the immune system

Treat insomnia

Relieve depression

Relax nerves and migraines.

Certain properties that are present in Tila and responsible for these benefits include anti-seizure property, anti-inflammatory properties, anti-cancer properties, anticonvulsant properties, neuroprotective properties, antispasmodic properties, to mention but a few. It works wonders on the gallbladder and liver too.

30. URTILA OIL

Urtila oil extracted from the nettle plant is used as a hair conditioner and to support oil production in the scalp.

31. VALERIAN

Origin: Asia, Europe

Valerian is used as a sedative. İt has anticonvulsant, antidepressant, and antianxiety properties. It relieves one who takes it of hysteria, anxiety, headache, nervousness, and exhaustion. Valerian also strengthens and relaxes the walls of the uterus.

32. YELLOW DOCK

Origin: Africa, Western Asia, Europe

Yellow Dock, especially the root works wonders as an antimicrobial, anti-inflammatory, analgesic, and antioxidant herb. It enhances the production of bile that aids the digestion of fats and improves the movement of the bowel in order to cleanse the digestive tract. Yellow Dock is called a blood purifier because it is a liver, lymphatic system, and gallbladder cleanser.

33. YOHIMBE

Origin: Western and Central Africa

Yohimbe fights against obesity, depression, and has the ability to enhance the libido. Due to its property in sexuality, it is used to reverse erectile dysfunction and increase sexual desires. This is essentially effective in females. Yohimbe herb is made from the bark of the tree. It is in ground form. The active ingredient in Yohimbe is the Yohimbine which can also be synthesized and sold as a more concentrated extract, but this is not recommended for usage. The bark of the Yohimbe plant that contains the Yohimbine ingredient naturally is less effective, compared to the synthesized form, but it is safer. This does not mean that the Yohimbine in the natural bark is not effective. It is very strong, and just a little amount is capable of increasing libido well.

34. DANDELION GREENS

The dandelion green is considered as a weed by a majority of people, but it is highly valued, alkalizing, and nutritious. Aside these, they are known to be anti-carcinogenic too. Dandelion leaves are great for salads or even as a tea. Their roots are helpful in treating kidney stones.

35. GARLIC

In a similar vein, garlic is anti-carcinogenic and highly alkalizing. It has been used for various purposes, which includes: antifungal, antiviral, and anti-parasitic treatments. It has its best alkaline level when it is fresh.

36. WHEATGRASS

Wheatgrass isn't far-fetched. It is just young wheat plants that are crushed, juiced, and used for medicinal purposes. It is highly alkalizing and has been used against certain health conditions such as gout, inflammation, cancer, etc.

37. CAYENNE PEPPER

Cayenne pepper is used as food and as medicine. It is eaten fresh and is used to treat pains, headaches, etc.

Amazingly, we have been through a lot of lessons just in this chapter. We have discussed exhaustively various herbs and supplements, their origin and precautions to taking them. Be careful to know that this book is in no way a substitute for your medical professional. Consult your doctor as often as possible and let him know, at each of your decisions and choices before you even enact them.

CHAPTER 07

HEALTH CONDITIONS IMPROVED BY THE ALKALINE

In the previous chapter, we have explained the herbs and supplements. You should go through their dosage, usage, and application. You must draw on these natural things in such a way that you get the best for optimum health attainment. They are very much available around you, although it is not everything that is food-related –as you must have known. In this chapter, we will move to certain health conditions that could be improved by the alkaline diet. We have not lost the aim of this book; providing optimum health attainment and maintenance through pH. We will explore the alkaline diet in a bid to teaching you how to improve health conditions. It isn't that you have health conditions but rather that you would be able to control them when they come around. In fact, with good knowledge of them, you would be able to apply this knowledge to people around you but do not forget to do so under medical supervision.

The alkaline diet is a meal plan advised by alternative medicine practitioners to help individuals maintain a healthy life, treat and prevent diseases. By meal plan, it is that they are a certain class of foods put to work together. Again, don't be too scared as these diets aren't meant to give you a particular pattern of food class to be consumed. The main thing is that you should see them as a guide to maintain good pH level and invariably optimum health attainment. The proponent advice that individuals consume more of fruits, low acid foods, seeds, legumes and vegetables and less of processed foods, fish, coffee, alcohol, soda, and high-fat dairy product. With scientific studies showing that alkaline diet improves the health, although disagreeing with the proposition that these meals play a role in the control of the pH level of the body, it can be shown without doubt that the alkaline diet improves health conditions and can be seen as an alternative to production of medications for many health conditions. The alkaline diet keeps emphasizing the need to consume plant-based foods. These plants based foods are moderately low in sodium but high in vitamins and minerals. Attributed to alkaline diets are benefits such as decreasing the risk of diseases due to the nutrients, antioxidants, and fiber it contains.

Although not totally correct in the way the proponents of the Alkaline diet theory put it forth, it is worthy of note that the diet plan encourages the consumption of certain meals which play a vital role in maintaining healthy conditions and it also shuns or reduces the intake of certain meals whose consumption might be detrimental. The meal plan for the alkaline diet should contain 80 percent of alkalizing food and 20 percent acid-forming food. For the purpose of this book, the ways alkaline diet helps to improve health conditions are discussed below;

ALKALINE DIET AND THE KIDNEY

Before we examine how the alkaline diet helps the kidney, we will need to know the organ and its role. The kidney plays an important role in ensuring that there is the regulation of the blood pH level, this it does, by removing excess substances that can make the blood acidic or alkaline. Also, the kidney is one of the organs necessary in homeostasis processes. Blood with a low pH level is said to be acidic, a condition which is known as acidosis and is fatal, so much that it calls for immediate medical attention. This is a crucial health condition relating to the organ mentioned here. Since the blood's normal pH is alkaline, and there is a need to ensure that the pH is kept constant (between 7.35 to 7.45) in order to avoid a low pH or a higher pH, by the kidney, there is a need to pay much attention to what one consumes as diets have been shown that the food an individual eats influences the amount of acid in the body.

It has been proven that for individuals with kidney disease, it becomes difficult for the kidney to maintain homeostasis, hence, the need for a high alkaline containing diet, in order to help such individuals balance their pH levels. Don't forget that homeostasis is important because it is the regulation of body temperature. Good adherence to the alkaline diet will enhance the combat against the health condition relating to lack of body temperature control.

Also, at the later stage of kidney diseases, the affected individuals need to limit their potassium intake; hence, a need for high alkaline containing diet. This is because when potassium is controlled, the exposure of the kidney to certain unfavorable condition for the infection of diseases such as gall stone could be very high. Meanwhile, when you maintain the alkaline diet plan given, you could elude such condition and move towards the attainment of optimum health condition.

Alkaline diet boosts Vitamin Absorption, preventing Magnesium Deficiency

In health conditions relating to deficiency in certain vitamin absorption, you will need to take in much food classes with a high rate of magnesium. This is because, for so many enzymatic activities and proper body metabolism, an increase in magnesium is necessary. In actuality, magnesium also activates Vitamin D, which is important in the immune and endocrine system function. The immune system, which is primarily needed for combating diseases, must be maintained all the time. In addition, the endocrine function for the overall body metabolism needs enough magnesium too. Everything needed to combat all of the health conditions could be controlled using the alkaline diet plan. Little wonder, the deficiency of magnesium may result in muscle pains, sleeplessness, heart complications, etc. therefore, an increased amount of magnesium, which can be got from Alkaline diet, is vital for health and vitality.

PROMOTING WEIGHT LOSS

Among many ladies are the desires to maintain a good weight. Although very many processes are involved in reducing weight, using the alkaline diet is one of the primary ways. By and large, losing weight is the goal of many individuals. However, it is a known fact that losing weight is dependent on the number of calories consumed in relation to the number of calories burned. Diets low in fat have been proven to help in weight loss, and physical activity in conjunction with a healthy diet also plays a vital role in weight loss. With lots of calories burned, it is very much easier to promote weight loss using the alkaline diet plan.

Primarily, alkaline diets are known to contain low calories, so, it helps people to lose weight. You have gone through chapter three that listed the kinds of alkalizing foods that could be consumed. To promote weight loss, you shouldn't bank on only exercises. Instead, watch the class of food you consume more and increase the food class with low calories.

HELP YOU MAINTAIN A HEALTHY WEIGHT

Obesity can be prevented, controlled, and dealt with by consuming less of acid-forming foods and more of alkaline-forming foods. This is possible because alkaline-forming foods decrease the level of leptin and inflammation that alters your hunger and fat-burning abilities. Did you know that alkaline-forming foods are anti-inflammatory and therefore gives it a chance to achieve normal leptin level? The normalized level of leptin will make you feel satisfied once you've eaten the number of calories you need.

ROLE IN CANCER

Alkaline diet plan plays a vital role in having cancer. This is because with meals low in acid-producing elements being the proposition upon which the alkaline diet theory is based –although without much scientific backing –it has been seen that individuals who consume meals high in the alkaline stand a lower risk of cancer than individuals who consume high acid containing meals. Once the level of cancer risk has been reduced by not consuming much acid-forming food classes, you are sure that getting optimum health is sure. The fact that your attention is a little bit drawn away from high acid-forming food makes it easier to have a low chance of having cancer.

LOWERING CHRONIC PAIN AND INFLAMMATION

Research has shown that there is a link between an alkaline diet and reduced levels of chronic pains. Acidosis, which is the accumulation of excess acid in the body leading to pH imbalance, has been found to be a contributing factor to joint pains, muscle and back pains, headaches and even menstrual symptoms. According to a study by the society for minerals and trace elements in Germany, it was discovered that after about four weeks of administration of alkaline supplements to patients with chronic back pains, 76 out of 82 were found to have noted a significant decrease in pain as measured using the "Arhus low back pain rating scale."

PREVENTING HEART DISEASE

Poor nutrition and low activity levels have been implicated in the cause of heart disease according to research carried out in 2010 in the United States of America. As the alkaline diet may increase the level of growth hormones (although the research was inconclusive), it is an established fact that growth hormones support body composition and lowers heart disease risk factors.

Since the alkaline diet is known to contain low acid-producing elements and minimal calories, it plays an important role in maintaining healthy body weight, thereby reducing the risk of cardiovascular diseases.

INCREASING GROWTH HORMONE LEVEL

The alkaline diet has been suggested to improve growth hormone level, as some proponents argue that a better heart rate is a prerequisite for having an improved growth hormone level, a role which has been linked to the consumption of alkaline-producing foods.

Reports suggest that an improved level of growth hormones promotes proper brain functioning and also improve the overall quality of life. The total full functioning of the brain will create good and sound mental health. This will indirectly affect overall health status. Good yield to the alkaline diet plan will afford you all these advantages.

Although the research about alkaline diets improving growth hormone level hasn't been well proven scientifically, however, there isn't much research to prove that they don't play any role as regards improving growth hormone level. In other words, this doesn't totally nullify their importance in the enhancement of hormones in the body.

ROLE IN PREVENTING OSTEOPOROSIS

Osteoporosis, a disease in which weakened bones increase the chances of having broken bones, a condition common among the elderly and females, is proven to be a major risk factor for fractures. Some proponents share the conviction that the alkaline diet reduces the amount of calcium lost out in the urine and that this lowers the risk of osteoporosis. However, scientific research doesn't really agree with this proposition.

Eating much fruits and vegetables may increase the general well-being of bones, and alkaline-rich foods serve this purpose.

PROTECTS BONE DENSITY.

In the total functioning of the muscles in the body, certain minerals are essential. It is a known fact that minerals are important in bone structure and development. The general protection of the body given by the muscles is carried out basically by the minerals. All these minerals could be supplied by using the alkaline diet plan. It is not that other food class wouldn't give these minerals, but proper monitoring will guarantee the areas of strength and weakness once there is a problem in metabolism. In other words, it will be easier to trace any form of alteration in the health conditions of the body with good adherence to the alkaline diet.

These minerals, such as calcium, magnesium, phosphate, to mention but a few, are essential for building strong bones and maintaining a good muscle mass. An alkaline diet plays a role in balancing the ratios of the minerals and also helping in the production of growth hormones and absorption of vitamins that protect the bones from other chronic diseases.

It has been proven that the more you consume alkalizing fruits and vegetables, the more protected you are from bone problems such as a decreased bone strength, which consequently leads to a weakening, and muscle wasting, as seen in the elderly, medically referred to as Sarcopenia.

In summary, the alkaline diet, despite its nonconformity with many scientific research results, is no doubt a diet that poses so many merits when consumed, as it plays various important roles in the maintenance of the body's structural and functional integrity.

Although, their roles in preventing or treating certain conditions have not been well defined, however, it is seen that they still play a role in the treatment of certain situations like cancer, cardiovascular diseases, and others.

Also, scientific research never proved or judged that alkaline diets are bad nor any less beneficial, hence, for those on the alkaline diet, it is a win-win situation, because away from the acid-alkaline theory about food, a diet rich in fresh fruits and vegetables is going to have amazing benefits to your overall health.

In this chapter, we have explained that there are certain health conditions that alkaline diet could be used to solve. That is, apart from giving optimum health status through the controlling of the acidity of the body, one enjoys control of some health conditions. These health conditions could be at any point in time, and the knowledge could be applied to friends around. The basic way is to maintain an alkaline diet plan. With this plan, you will be able to consume certain food class in a specific pattern to combat the health conditions. Proper attention needs to be taken to the nutrients rather than the food itself for full applications of this chapter. In the next chapter, we will move forward to something a little bit outside, the consumption of food. Stay tuned!

CHAPTER 08

THE ACIDIC EFFECT OF STRESS, ANGER AND NEGATIVE THINKING ON THE BODY

You should know that what you eat is quite responsible for how you feel. The food you are eating might be the cause of your depressed state. And consequently, the way you feel will affect your overall health. It is clear that feelings could be subjected to lots of things that make them temporal. That is, what you feel now might change in the next seconds. However, knowing the causes of these feelings is crucial. They are actually altered by our daily activities. Based on the fact that everyone surely has routines, the effect they have on the body determines the way feel on a daily basis. This makes it crucial to examine them and their effects on the body.

Certain foods trigger certain hormones in the body, and this is the need for watching whatever it is we eat. Most people are too busy with work and life, and in the same vein, do not eat a good and nutritious diet. Your hormones are fundamental in your body as the brain communicates with other parts of the body by the help of your hormones. Your hormones can be in a state not so right termed as Hormonal imbalance. This can be as a result of so many reasons like chronic stress levels, anger, and negative thinking. It has been observed in older men and women where there is an increase or drastic decrease in the level of estrogen, cortisol, or testosterone. In most of these cases, medications might just conceal the symptoms and not deal with the problem directly, but with a right understanding of natural remedies such as having to eat the right kind of food, these conditions are improved. Our Acid-Alkaline diet is hormone-friendly.

The diet, food, and nutrients you provide your body with is what fuels your system into producing the necessary and needed hormones and all (note that diet is not the only factor as heredity can be a major.) it is essential that the right kind of food and the right proportion of food is to be given to your body system so as make the best out of it. If your diet does not supply the right building block for hormonal formation and function, stress hormones are produced as the first line of action because those are quite essential for survival. Therefore, during chronic fatigue and stress, you may have fluctuated hormone levels and imbalance. Note that stress can be from various sources such the emotional, psychological, and even physical which involves not eating appropriately, having excess acid in the body, having an infection or disease, etc. So when stress is mentioned, it does not speak only of sleeplessness and being worked out.

Your hormones and you!

There are so many hormones in the body and can be referred to as the body's chemical messengers. These hormones are produced in what is called the endocrine glands, and there are quite a number of them, i.e., Adrenal, Pineal, Hypothalamus, Thyroid, Ovaries, pituitary gland, to mention just a few. Some of the various hormones produced by them are:

- CORTISOL

Cortisol affects your alertness, sleep, fat storage, etc., and can affect weight, fertility, cognitive health, and mood in both male and female.

- PROGESTERONE

This is one of the female sex hormones. It regulates the Uterus lining in women and acts as a counterbalance to estrogen, which is also another sex hormone in females. It can affect emotional health, sleep, and mood.

- ESTROGEN

Like discussed in the hormone mentioned above, it is a female sex hormone, and it is of three major types: Estrone, Estradiol, and Estriol. They all can affect fertility, menstruation, and menopause in women.

• TESTOSTERONE

Like estrogen, testosterone is a sex hormone produced by both men and women, but it is produced more in men. Testosterone is responsible for energy, sex drive, alertness, muscle mass, strength, and fertility. A level lower than the norm of testosterone can cause sexual dysfunction. This is why there is a need for hormonal balance.

• INSULIN

This hormone is secreted by the pancreas and helps transport blood sugar (glucose) into various cells for use and into certain tissues for storage, when in excess in the blood. This hormone must be kept in total balance because an increase in insulin level can lead to medical conditions such as diabetes, weight gain, reproductive problems, to mention but a few.

• LEPTIN

Leptin works with hunger and satisfaction signaling. It tells the brain when you are hungry and when exactly you are full. It also helps note how the body burns fat.

These aforementioned mentioned hormones are just a few among so many. But noting their benefits and purpose should give you a better understanding has to why they must be kept in optimum balance. You cannot afford to let the levels of these hormones sway to and fro as this can endanger your health and even life. These hormones are the basics of you. They stand to should what you are made of alive. They can bring about death too when not in proper array and proportion.

Don't forget that this book centers on giving you tips to maintaining sound health by considering the food types you consume. This, in return, specifies the pH level of all the food. How do factors such as stress, anger, negative thinking, etc. contribute to alkalizing your body? Note that the bottom line is to help you live optimum health; this is why this chapter has been incorporated in order to know other things that affect health status aside food.

The truth remains that thoughts and emotions are vitalities in health. How? Emotions that are expressed or experienced without much issues and thoughts tend to slip without altering our health. But fearful and negative emotions are capable of zapping the body of its energy, mentally and in all spheres, and this can lead to further health problems. Certainly, poorly-managed emotions are not good for health. Everything surrounding negative emotions most likely results in depression. The thing is, when one is mentally depressed based on lack of self-confidence or fear of failure and future, it will surely affect the overall optimum health status. This is because thinking right and acting at the right time will be altered. In fact, one could innocently do what is detrimental to oneself. This is part of the reasons for this chapter; understanding other external key factors that could contribute to optimum health status.

Bad emotions and negative feelings are also capable of creating stress, which will destabilize the body's chemicals and hormones found in the brain, thereby leading to damage to the immune system. Stress, according to science, can decrease our lifespan. This is possible because stress is capable of shortening our DNA's telomeres (the endpoints of DNA strands), causing us to age more quickly. Stress is one of the things that could damage the brain. When one is stressed out without getting enough sleep, it will be difficult to carry out adequate metabolism. This will, in turn, affect health status. Though everyone does many things that stress them out, monitoring stress, and doing the necessary things to avoid, it is crucial. With lots of stress, dementia could be developed, especially in adult women. Of course, the strength of most ladies can't be equalized with gentlemen. Thus the time they are stressed out varies. Women need to take of this in order to know the extent they could work and the type of jobs they can do at a time.

Anger, especially when poorly managed, is

associated with having caused health conditions such as hypertension (also known as High Blood Pressure), infections, digestive disorders, and other cardiovascular diseases. It has been established that the number of veins that are stressed during anger is many. Sometimes, anger could be a state of mind at a time. This means that one doesn't get triggered to anger by external forces, rather the annoyance is just without source. What is actually happening is that you are going through lots of thoughts with which you barely have solutions. Overthinking and overreacting to certain situations could have been the cause of this "internal" anger. When you are angry, your mind is far from the immediate environment to the extent of you causing yourself harms unknowingly. It could as well be that you are faced with lots of challenges or choices which you can't but face; this could lead to anger.

To manage stress, anger, and negative thinking,

I recommend these exercises:

- YOGA

Yoga helps you manage your overall well-being and comportment. Especially in ladies, it is known to increase strength, mood, and concentration and muscle tone. It enhances body posture and flexibility. It is perfect for managing stress and improving your breathing ability. It has been proven too that weight loss is possible with yoga, although the rate is slightly low relative to other aerobic exercises. Aside all of the merits mentioned above of yoga, it also has been known to be an effective exercise that relieves joint pains and disorders while strengthening and stretching the joints.

- MEDITATION

The importance of meditation cannot be over-emphasized. It is known for improvement in creative thinking, stress levels, energy, and even success. Meditation changes our brain (I do not mean you get a new pair!) but the neurons and cells are kept healthy, constantly making new connections and cutting off the old based on the response it receives. Meditation is associated with improvement in a lot of psychological areas that include: stress, cognitive function, addiction, anxiety, depression, etc.

- WALKING IN NATURE

Another exciting exercise that immensely helps in fitness is walking in nature. It has been proven to have mental benefits while reducing the risk of depression and Improving your fitness level by building a strengthened heart. Going to tourist centers is one of the ways of managing stress. Very many people move to where they could see nature because seeing them gives the brain a kind of sustainable relaxation. Actually, walking in nature and observing its natural ways of moving around could enhance mental health.

This is a psychological effect on the manner of thinking. This is why people take time to utilize their vacations and holidays very well. It has even been proven that mild exercises such as walking, especially in nature or around places you love are a fantastic therapy in skin tone, weight loss, and healthy nerves.

- LISTENING TO MUSIC, ESPECIALLY CLASSICAL

Music is art, and art is music. It is entertaining and has an amazing therapeutic effect on its listener. Not all types of music are appealing, as too loud ones can be distasteful and distracting. Good classical music helps improve memory, attention, coordination, and brain development. Music heals. It causes the body to release endorphins in response to pains. It is relaxing and softens breathing and heartbeat, reducing blood pressure too. In so many parts of the world, music has been recognized as one of the means of relaxing the brain to enhance body metabolism. This is one of the ways of managing stress in the body.

There are other ways to cope with stress, which include; reading, taking a long walk, getting a massage, and lots more. Concerning reading, when you are stressed or angry, you could get a book that could distract your thoughts away from the situations around. This will not only keep your thoughts from other negative thoughts of the stress consequences but also lighten up your mood as you imagine your presence in the plot of the story.

As regards taking a long walk, you could manage stress by having an intentional walk from stipulated time duration consistently. This is a form of passive body exercise that stimulates body metabolism and promote mental health. The effect of exercises on health can't be overemphasized. The body will regain enough strength after the exercise. The sweating through walking will help in removing harmful substances in the body.

Based on massage, the body receives adequate relief from stress by going through massage. There are different types of body massage, but their effect is almost the same; providing the body with sound mental health. Certain harmful substances in the body too will be removed with good body massage. In a bid to manage stress, get a good massage. Note that it doesn't have to be done by experts, you could do it on your own by relaxing your body and massaging all the joints.

Over time, it has been noticed that mental and emotional stress creates more acids in the body. It results in the production of lactic acid, which, when in excess, is toxic to the body. A remedy to too much and too fast production of lactic acid is that rest must be taken, exercise often, and the consumption of alkaline water is advised. A common and most ignored aspect of stress is dehydration. According to research, 80% of Americans are dehydrated. Dehydration is noted as the number one trigger of fatigue during the day. And a 2% drop in the body water can reduce an athlete's performance and even lead to memory loss. But ten glasses of water, daily, can significantly ease 80% of people with back and joint pains, five glasses can reduce breast cancer by 78%, colon cancer by 45% and bladder cancer by 50%.

Water is an essential substance in sustaining all forms of life. It moistens all tissues and protects internal and external organs. It also dissolves nutrients and minerals, even toxins that are stuck in the body, veins, and passages. It helps in heat regulation, joint lubrication, and also assists in the transport of nutrients and oxygen to various cells. It is a popular saying that you need to drink about half of your weight in ounce water daily. The essentiality of water in healthy living can't be overemphasized. One could survive longer, just taking only water compare to what happens with eating.

CHAPTER 09

HOW TO SUSTAIN HIGH ENERGY LEVELS USING THE ALKALINE DIET.

Do you think you are living your life to the fullest? Health-wise, do you realize you are not using up all of the potentials you have inside you? Do you even feel really incapable and assume aging is the reason? If not, as perfect and as much as you utilize all of your potentials, imagine if just about half of that strength is what you have now. Don't you think life would be better with much more strength, perfection and potential?

So many people are deprived of health and wellness due to certain diseases and health condition that are most likely as a result of poor feeding habits and pH imbalance. But it is a pity that so many attributes all of this ailments and weaknesses to old age and the aging phenomenon. A lot of us encounter stress and are faced with all of life's challenges, which, with full force, keeps us pressured on every side. With all of these, maximizing the goodness of life and feeling healthy is still very far away.

It's disheartening. I know! As much as we now can spot a problem, we cannot stop at that, an answer that provides a solution is what we should consider next.

I am happy to tell you that this is the way to rejuvenation. Aren't you ready to understand what it takes to feel good and energized? Do you want to enjoy every moment of life in health, strength and perfect wellness? If yes, keep on reading. And if no, I love you, so much, and I do not want this to pass you by, therefore keep on reading. You will discover life-changing facts in this chapter that would help you.

Just as it's been a major focus in this book, diet plays an extremely important role in the life of all living beings. We are not disputing the fact that other factors can contribute to weakness and health problems, but an important one is a diet, yes, diet. It is no mere saying that "we are what we eat." When you eat better, you live better.

Certain steps that we see as small and insignificant in life are usually the most important ones. A change in your diet can make an immense difference in your whole life, either for better or for worse. A diet that is alkaline and acid balance is great and really helpful in regaining energy level and in living life fully. It is cheap and easy to abide by. It does not employ compulsion, restriction, and other exhausting steps, like other diet types do. The alkaline diet is capable of undoing damages that unhealthy eating habits and yo-yo dieting have done to your body over the years, and re-energizing your body by giving it the proper nutrition it requires. The main goal off this diet type is to help both men and women have a healthier body and an active mind.

To get started with the alkaline diet, it is advised that you see your doctor. The alkaline diet super-food list has been provided in this book earlier. Get acquainted with the list and make provisions for the ones you can afford and are available in grocery stores at your area. A help with classifying has been done on the super-food list in this book too, you can also write or print this food list out and have it pinned to your notice board or on your refrigerator. This should help. With this chart and list, you can plan your meal perfectly well, and you can appropriately monitor your intake of acid-forming and alkaline-forming foods.

Oh, NO! Did I mention that? I haven't said alkaline diet involves eating mundane, boring, or even irritating foods. Hell, no! I know you will be salivating at the sight of certain delicious and yummy delicacies that you do not know about yet. In fact, I personally find alkaline recipes as delicious, easy, and not to forget, healthy too.

A higher energy level means a higher and more efficient body and mind. And with great efficiency in body and mind, the way you feel is improved, and your productivity is enhanced.

Have you ever drawn a link between what you eat and how you feel? I must say that you are a genius to have thought in that pattern. From the evidence, and recent researches, it is suggested that there is a link between what we eat and how we feel. A healthy diet that is rich in fruits, whole grains, and vegetables is said to boost mood and fight depression. Junk food and processed foods are likely to lower moods and increase depression. Psychologically, the mood is known to be highly subjective and can be influenced by our perception and the beliefs we hold, individually. This point and other factors are not neglected as they can sway the mind and mood, but as important as they are, diet is also a factor. The diet factor is not just inferred and said, quite an amount of studies has been done to monitor the effect of diet on the mood, overtime.

Note that, not a single food is responsible for a change in the mood or mind's activity, but a routine/diet is.

An increase or decrease in the blood sugar level can also influence your mood over a short period of time. Your consumption of processed foods can alter your mood too, though it is difficult to point out a particular substance that affects the mood in processed food because there are so many components in processed foods. It has been said by Dr. Felice Jacka of the University of Deakin, that certain unhealthy food components are known to (from thorough research in animal studies) affect the brain directly and the hippocampus is most negatively affected: the site for mood regulation and other things and processes. There is and will be a great improvement in your mood once you begin to avoid processed foods. In fact, an overall shift to health and wellness will be noted once you move away from processed food towards whole foods.

CHAPTER 10

HOW TO EXERCISE WHEN FOLLOWING THE ALKALINE DIET

By now, you are familiar with the alkaline diet, right? Amazing! You sure must have learned a whole lot from this book. You now know that the basics of the alkaline diet are that you eat less of acidic (acid-forming) foods and more of alkaline foods. This principle is to stabilize the body's pH and allow the normal function of processes in the body. Just for the records, getting alkaline extends not only to diet but even to exercise.

Did you know that not all exercises are alkalizing and oxygenating to your body? Most of the exercises you carry out are highly acid-forming! Though you presume you are getting the most out of your daily workout, it might be the reason you are prone to unhealthy conditions and even weight gain.

Apart from your devotion to eating what is right, did you know that your workout can be a factor contributing to the build-up of acids in your system? Not all workouts support and promote alkalinity. The workouts that promote alkalinity are aerobics that builds cardio and controlled breathing. These aerobics increase the flow of oxygen to the heart, muscles, lungs, blood, and cells. This flow helps to detoxify the tissues and provide the necessary circulation of nutrients by the help of oxygen. Acid-Alkaline diet is so encompassing as it understands the need even when it comes to exercise. You can't get rid of excess acid-forming foods and still build up acid in your body system through the kind of exercises you do. That is why this chapter is written. To make you understand what kind of exercises are that are best for you. You could call them "Acid-Alkaline Exercises" ... because they matter in your quest and search for optimum health and balance.

Here is a list of the good aerobics that would aid your health and not alter your routine. In following the alkaline diet, therefore, you must consider the 'alkaline exercise' too.

- JUMPING

The first on the list of exercises that actually works is Jumping. It works in squeezing out toxins and poisons from the cells, tissues and lymphatic system. It is a wash and detox form of exercise. When you jump around, you breathe deeply, and sufficient oxygen is provided to your respiratory system. It is super-efficient because it deals with the fundamental level of life, which is the cell, and when the cells are healthy, there is an assurance of an overall healthy body and life. This exercise is the most powerful exercise to keep your cells healthy. It is fun, increases metabolism and circulation, and helps you burn fat.

- SWIMMING

Swimming is also an aerobic workout, though not as efficient and with low impact, it works wonders on the lungs. Your breathing is more efficiently done, because in swimming, you breathe in the fresher air and carbon dioxide is expelled graciously. Aside from the fact that swimming helps in reducing the production of lactic acid in your body, its calming and relaxing effect when you are submerged in water has been proven to relieve chronic stress. It is the best way to relax after a long day. It is great at dealing with stress and fatigue. It is quite amazing and soothing to sit in the pool, viewing nature, and playing around with friends and family.

- YOGA

You cannot sustain alkalinity entirely alone by just diet. Remember, balance is what we crave, it is essential to incorporate balanced exercises too of which YOGA comes first. Yoga is founded on the principle that the body and mind must be united; when you exercise your body, your mind is incorporated too. Yoga relieves stress. Stress, as you've known, is a factor that can build up acid in the body. Yoga also encourages deep breathing, just like swimming. You should know that deep breathing is a form of detoxification and hence an alkalizing practice.

- TAI CHI

Last but not least, TAI CHI is also a known beneficial and healthy workout. Tai Chi has been in existence for about 2000 years now. It is known for a variety of benefits such as increased flexibility, improved sleep, improved balance, decrease in stress, muscle, and joint pain. In fact, recent research has shown that in a trial of 100, 85% noted a reduction in blood pressure.

Therefore, Tai Chi is efficient in improving cardiovascular functions and lowering blood pressure.

In summary, more than any other food or drink, stress is of greater harm to your body system. Practice tai chi, yoga, swimming, and meditation. Be sure to practice deep breathing because most of the acid in your body (carbon dioxide) is passed out through the lungs. Fresh foods are still very much available in the marketplace. Eat more raw foods and farm produce. Make sure to exercise daily, cooking more at home than eating out.

Try intermittent fasting and see how it makes you feel. I believe intermittent fasting and the alkaline diet can give you amazing health results when applied together. This will be further discussed in the next chapter of this book.

CHAPTER 11

FASTING ON THE ALKALINE DIET

THE ANCIENT WISDOM OF FASTING AND WHAT DOES SCIENCE SAY ABOUT IT

When you decide to consciously and voluntarily not eat food for a length of time, that is fasting. This voluntary abstinence is, of course, for a specified time. Fasting is seen as a spiritual practice in many religions all over the world, including Islam, Christianity, even Buddhism. It has been used therapeutically for many conditions too. In fact, fasting is noted to be one of the oldest therapies in medicine because it has been used for thousands of years. It is recommended as a healing method and preventive measure by many great doctors of which are

• HIPPOCRATES

He is the father of modern medicine. He believed that fasting is a mechanism that allows the body to heal itself up in times needed.

- ## PARACELSUS

Paracelsus is another great healer who believed in fasting and worked in the western tradition. In one of his writings, he said that fasting is the greatest remedy; it is the physician within.

A renowned healing system called the "Ayurvedic medicine" also advocates fasting as a major treatment, and this it has done for a very long time. To mention but a few, many other great spiritual leaders like Buddha, Jesus, and Mohammed, fasted for mental, physical, and spiritual strength. Also, to promote peace, it was noted that the famous Indian leader, Mahatma Gandhi fasted for a period of 21 days.

In Europe, fasting is used for treatment for years now. Even spas and treatment centers in Germany, Russia, and Sweden use fasting for medical purposes under supervision. Fasting is also popular in America and has served as an alternative medicine for several decades. In detoxification and detoxification programs that are based on the principle that illnesses and health conditions are caused by the buildup of toxins in the body, fasting is usually the center of all therapy.

WHY THEN SHOULD YOU FAST?

The benefits of fasting cannot be overemphasized. In this chapter, we will discuss a few of these benefits and see the reasons why we should fast.

1. Fasting works for illnesses and almost all chronic condition. For allergies, digestive disorders, high cholesterol, diabetes, and headaches, fasting has been known to relieve and even cure them.

2. Fasting is great for losing weight.

3. It is an efficient way and trusted method in detoxification.

4. Fasting, aside from other curative purposes, is known to for preventive measures because it helps in increasing overall health, vitality and helps the body build resistance to diseases.

Fasting is just when the intake of food that is eating is stopped temporarily. It is more like you are giving your body and internal organs, especially the digestive tract which is the most prone to threats due to intake of bacteria, toxins, and virus from the immediate environment through the gut, and system a break from hard work. In the process, a certain amount of calories is burnt, and toxic substances stored in the body are expelled.

The whole process that occurs in your stomach is that when food is eaten

· It is broken down in the intestines

· Then it travels via the blood to the liver (from basic biology, the liver is the largest organ of the body and also and thee site for detoxification.)

· The liver, in return, breaks down the food substances passed to it and then removes the toxins present in the food.

Now when food is entirely and continuously taken in, the liver does a whole lot of work removing toxin from the food and particularly storing it in other parts of the body. So, when you fast, the liver is freed from duty and therefore has the time to detoxify other organs of the body and heal them as well.

SCIENCE OF FASTING.

The science of fasting is a handy and important study that has proven its efficiency and potency over the years. It is known for its immense health benefits that include longevity of life.

This fasting is seen in various forms and practices. It is otherwise known as the time-restricted feeding, whereby the number of caloric intake is reduced at a certain period of time. This period of time is usually not less than eight hours though it can be more than 12 hours per day.

Based on certain scientists, fasting can be:

TIME-RESTRICTED FEEDING

It was by the Scientist, Satchidananda Panda

According to him, Time-restricted fasting (TRF) is the act of limiting your calorie intake for a specified length of time between 8-12 hours per day.

INTERMITTENT CALORIE RESTRICTION

This one was by the scientist Michelle Harvie.

Calorie restriction, like the name implies, involves that you reduce your calorie intake level by half to about 800 or 1000 calories. It advocates that a two-day calorie restriction must occur in your diet every week. It is most times referred to as intermittent fasting.

PERIODIC FASTING AND FASTING MIMICKING DIET

Valter Longo is the scientist behind this work.

In this model, what is required is that one limits calories intake between three and five days so that body cells can take from the glucose (glycogen, which is then stored form of glucose in the liver and other organs)

INTERMITTENT FASTING ON THE ALKALINE DIET

In the alkaline diet, just as we have established that it extends to all spheres, even exercise. It is important to note that not only does the right food and right exercise matter, but food must also be eaten in the right and appropriate pattern.

Therefore, intermittent fasting is not about the diet but the pattern of eating. It involves systematically scheduling your meals inappropriate manners and way so that you can have the best out of them. Intermittent fasting does not in any way change the kind of foods you eat, but it changes when you eat them. So, in the alkaline diet, having intermittent fasting will mean eating alkaline-forming foods that balance the body's pH in a manner that sequentially allows you to get the best out them.

It is a great way to cut down on your calories intake and allow the food you just consume give its best to your body system. It is notably, a great way to keep the muscle mass in place even while getting lean. It is an efficient way to get lean and lose significant weight, especially within a short period of time. You want to lose weight the right way and with ease? Just a moment and we'd be talking about that.

Intermittent fasting is perhaps the easiest way to get rid of bad and excess weight while keeping the good weight on. It requires some behavior change, though it might seem tedious at the start. Aren't you excited that intermittent fasting falls in the group of weight-loss activity that is easy to do yet powerful enough to make the difference?

NOW TO THE QUESTION 'HOW?'

How do you think intermittent fasting leads to fat loss? Could it be that the intermittent fast uses a knife on your body to curve the unhealthy you into the better version? No! First, you must understand basic concepts to know and understand how fasting works in weight loss. In biochemistry and food science study, we have concepts like fed state and fasted state, and just as the names imply, the fed state is that phase when your body is digesting and absorbing food that has just been consumed. This phase begins when you start to eat and lasts for as long as four to five hours after the meal. In that period, the foods are digested and absorbed. At this fed state, foods are broken down, and insulin is in high concentration or level, picking up the foods for storage. Therefore, it is very hard for the body system to burn fats.

After that period of time, the body is no longer processing any food. It is referred to as the post-absorptive state. The post-absorptive state lasts for about 8 to 12 hours after your meal, and thereafter, you enter into the fasted state. In this state, that is the fasted state. It is quite easier to burn fat because the insulin level is low. At the fed state, fats are inaccessible, but during the fasted state, the body has access to the fat stores and hence the possibility of burning them.

Now, the fasted state is not achieved until 12 hours after a meal, and because most of us eat meals and delicacies round the clock, it is rare, and our bodies are barely in that fasted state. It is therefore almost impossible to lose or burn fats. This is where intermittent fasting comes into play.

Intermittent fasting helps you lose weight even when you barely change what you eat. So with the alkaline diet, allowing the fasted state to burn fats is healthy enough and accompanies your perfect diet routine.

The Benefits of Intermittent Fasting

Intermittent fasting provides a wide range of health benefits but does not force one into any massive lifestyle change.

1. Fasting simplifies your day this is by reducing the number of meals you have to plan, prepare, and cook. An average person eats three times a day, but with intermittent fasting, you have one meal less to plan for and prepare. Isn't this an easy one?

2. Intermittent fasting has been proven to increase lifespan. Intermittent fasting works in burning the bad weights and help retain the good ones which strengthen your body and

increase life expectancy.

3. Intermittent fasting has been said to have a slight good in lowering the risk of cancer.

4. Fasting can help you lose weight. Fasting puts your body in a fat-burning state. This will help you lose weight easily and in no long time.

5. Intermittent fasting is much easier, productive, and easy to stick to in the long term. You can quickly adapt to the fasting routine.

HOW DO YOU GET STARTED?

It isn't a rigid start. There are different intermittent fasting schedules, and each produces different results. For the purpose of this book, we have three schedules explicitly outlined and explained. Read all three methods and choose the fasting schedule that is aligned with your goals.

1. Daily intermittent fasting

2. Weekly intermittent fasting

3. Alternate day intermittent fasting

You can choose which suits you and your lifestyle, work, and/or family.

DAILY INTERMITTENT FASTING

A well-known model that daily intermittent

fasting is that of Leangains. It is called Leangain's model. This model uses a 16- hours fast followed by an 8-hour eating period. This model was named after the originator, Martin Berkhan, who owned Leangains.com. The 8-hour eating time can start any time you are comfortable with, and it doesn't really matter when you start. Daily intermittent fasting is done every day, and this makes it very easy to get used to. If you considerably check your routine of eating, you will notice that you eat almost around the same time every day without even knowing it. All you need to do is get used to not eating some certain meals, and that will be easy.

IN SUMMARY,

- The fast is on for about sixteen hours, but about eight hours of the time, you most likely will be in bed because it is the night time.

- Your first meal for the new day will, therefore, be after these sixteen hours.

WEEKLY INTERMITTENT FASTING

Another brilliant way to get intermittent fasting done is by starting with the schedule once per week. This might not be so fast a weight-loss activity, but other benefits associated with fasting is attributed to this schedule too. For instance, when your last meal is lunch on Monday, you will fast till lunch on Wednesday while you enjoy every other day of the week. This schedule is flexible and still effective and beneficial though it is less likely to lose so much weight when using this schedule. This is ideal and perfect if you just want to keep fit and not lose so much weight. This schedule is most times advised after a long day of the festival or big holidays.

In other words, you are to fast for about 24 hours every week.

ALTERNATE DAY INTERMITTENT FASTING

Alternate day intermittent fasting incorporates longer fasting periods on alternating days throughout the week. That is, you are to start a 16-24hours fast and break the fast the next day'. This fast type, alternate day intermittent fasting schedule, allows you to eat at least one meal in a day. To explain that, let us say you are fasting for 24 hours, you could have your dinner on Tuesday night and fast till Wednesday night. So, on Thursday, you get to eat all three meals in a day but start the fasting cycle again for 24 hours after dinner on that Thursday.

This style is not adopted by many people but is used by some scientists for research and studies purpose.

This schedule makes you stay fasted for a longer period of time, so you are more 'fasted' than you are 'fed.' Hence this would increase the benefits of fasting. Honestly, the biggest barrier to getting started with this intermittent fasting is the mental barrier. It prevents people from fasting, assuming it is hard, but in the real sense, it's really not that hard to do in practice.

WHY YOU SHOULDN'T SEE INTERMITTENT FASTING AS HARD OR DIFFICULT.

It is crystal clear that fasting has been practiced by so many religious groups and for centuries now. Medically, it has been noted for health benefits and improvements over time. Therefore, fasting isn't a cumbersome activity that is just evolving. It has been in existence for years, people have been undergoing it, and it works.

Furthermore, you sure must have fasted without you knowing it. Can you recall when you actually forgot to take breakfast or were to engross in house chores and duties and resorted to a late brunch? Must you have slept at some nights without having dinner and then do not eat till about noon the next day? You have fasted for about 10 hours without you even knowing. It is not as difficult as you think. You can and have done it before.

INTERMITTENT FASTING FOR WOMEN

Just as it's been discussed in this book earlier, intermittent fasting talks more on WHEN to eat by introducing regular eating routines than WHAT to eat. This enhances weight loss, reducing your risk of heart diseases and diabetes. However, from recent research and studies, it has been suggested that intermittent fasting is not as beneficial for women like it is for men. Therefore, a better and modified system of the intermittent fasting is introduced.

Intermittent fasting is a pattern of eating that combines times and days of fasting and normal eating routine days. It includes the alternate days fast, 16 hours fast in a day, and about 24 hours fast in a week. All of these routines are collectively called intermittent fasting.

Several studies have provided shreds of evidence to confirm that intermittent fasting may affect men and women differently. Particular research showed that the blood sugar level control in women who undergo intermittent fasting worsens after three weeks of the routine. Another study narrates the story of women, who after they started the intermittent fasting, experienced changes in their menstrual cycles. All of these changes occur because the female body is highly sensitive to calorie intake and restriction.

A woman who fasts intermittently, or perhaps

for too long, has low-calorie intake which affects a part of the brain known as the hypothalamus. This then alters the secretion of the gonadotropin-releasing hormone that helps in the release of two reproductive hormones. When these two hormones are lacking and cannot communicate with the ovaries, the risk of irregular periods is increased, and this can be accompanied by infertility, and other health problems such as poor bone health.

Therefore, it is advised that women consider a modified approach to intermittent fasting that would incorporate shorter fasting times and fewer fasting days.

Listed below are five best forms and types of intermittent fasting for women.

1. Crescendo Method: this method of intermittent fasting allows one to fast for about 12-16 hours for two to three days a week. These fasting days must be nonconsecutive. It, instead, should be evenly spaced across the week.

2. Modified Alternate-Day fasting: this fast method allows you to fast on every other day aside the non-fasting days. On these non-fasting days, you are to eat normally as you would, perhaps three times a day. While you are allowed to consume 20-25% of your usual calorie intake on the fasting days.

3. Eat-stop-Eat: The Eat-stop-eat method is otherwise known as the 24hours protocol. It incorporates 24 hours full fast once or twice in a week. This can start with about 14-16 hours fast and gradually till it builds up but the maximum number of times a week for the woman must be two.

4. The fast diet: this method is otherwise called the 5:2 method. It restricts calorie intake to 25% of your usual consumption, which is about 500 calories for two days in a week and you get to eat normally for the other five days.

5. The Leangains method: this is otherwise called the 16/8 method. Here, you get to fast for 16hours a day and all calories for the next 8 hours. You could start with 14 hours fast till you eventually can have the 16 hours.

With all of these approaches listed, it is important to eat healthy and well during the fasting and the non-fasting days. And be sure to work with the approach you can tolerate and sustain in a long-term without having any negative health consequences.

Be sure to consult your doctor if you have any medical conditions and before trying the intermittent fasting.

CHAPTER 12

WEIGHT LOSS PITFALLS

It is a fact that when a diet is new to your body, your body might not know how best and correctly to respond to it. If the acid-alkaline is new to you and your body system, I mean if you've never undergone this, your body may not know the best way to respond initially. In fact, you might have negative feedbacks at the start like more weight gain, weak body, and reduced energy level, etc., but do not panic, your weight can fluctuate at times, it is normal. When you maintain the acid-alkaline balance, however, an amazing benefit is weight loss. When you feed on a healthy and natural diet, chances that you grow fat and chunky is very slim, although it is quite difficult to lose weight that you have gained over time. In this chapter, we will see obstacles to losing weight and how to overcome them.

To start with, when you go through a change in diet, your body gets notified and store up certain calories, a mechanism to help sustain the body in case of starvation. So for a start, look critically into your current diet and see if it is acid supporting or alkaline excessive or a balanced one. Once you have noted your diet, if it is not appropriate, that is if your diet isn't the balanced acid-alkaline diet and you have to get a change, then your body might show off certain weird developments in response to the change. This is because the body will have to adjust to the inflow of enzymes, alkaline-forming foods, and other healthy substances.

TIP: Be sure to drink plenty of water when you start the acid-alkaline diet. This is because water is essential to prevent stool retention. Make it slow and steady both with an intake of water and other alkaline foods. It is great to start small than push beyond your limit from the start.

Just so you'd know, a scale can be an amazing way to get to know your weight, but I know you do have heartaches when you realize you haven't lost as much as weight as you thought or that you have added weight. The scale cannot differentiate between the weight of your muscles, fats, nor fluid. It only measures that overall body weight, which is composed of the organs, bones, fluid, muscles, and fat. From previously explained fats in this book, you will know that shedding fluff and building lean muscles through aerobic exercises. Oftentimes, you do not know where you are going to because you have not figured out where you were and are now. Look back and discover how the former diets have failed.

Examine the approach you used then be sure to make a change. Though certain cogent reasons might be why you couldn't make it through the former diet you quitted, these are reasonable but do not assume to quit because of

- You feel it isn't and wouldn't work

- You got tired and bored with the whole process.

- You are scared

It is absolutely okay, as humans, to feel and get bored at a diet that restricts you and forces you to eat what you do not like. Thanks to the acid-alkaline diet that, fortunately, will not stop you from eating anything you love eating but would, rather, teach you what acids and acid-forming foods are and can do to your health. With this knowledge, it is much easier to let go of the bad foods.

In addition, the acid-alkaline diet is one you can keep doing for a lifetime. It isn't harmful. It is a perfect balance in the body. The standard American diet, abbreviated as SAD, is loaded with red meat, fast foods, and other trans fats. This diet, when in excess, gives a terribly high amount of unhealthy fats but the acid-alkaline diet, which emphasizes vegetables and natural ground foods provide healthy fats.

The link is that a high amount of acids in your body makes your body hold on to fat, even faster.

The little acid in your meal and then in your body is gotten rid of by metabolism and released in the urine. However, excess consumption of acid-forming foods makes your system clouded, and this is taken to the fat cells to be stored. We can illustrate this by saying that fat is a garage, and acid is a car parked in that garage. With enough space in the garage, so many cars are accommodated. This excess fat sums up and leads to one type of fat storage called the visceral fat. The visceral fat is that fat around your internal organ. This is not entirely due to the intake of acid-forming foods but also stress and hormonal fluctuations. It isn't easy to lose these fats, but neither is it impossible. All you need to do it decrease the amount of acid-forming foods you consume and start living stress-free.

SET GOALS

This isn't as most motivational speaking, the fact of life is that you are at the best way of achieving any goal as much as you plan and map out your way to achieve them, this includes weight loss.

When you start losing weight, it connotes that stored fats are liquefied and removed from your body. This process of losing weight is remarkable explained in three processes, which are

- Diet

- Exercise

- Overcoming obstacles

Diet has been properly addressed in this book, and so is exercise. Obstacles are most times under-diagnosed. These obstacles may seem minor, but they mean a lot and get in your way towards achieving weight loss. These obstacles may include

- A bad knee

- Soda addiction

- Veggie aversion etc.

So that your effort wouldn't be wasted, it is advised that you deal with these weaknesses, even before you begin this new lifestyle. To improve your rate of success, identify and get rid of your weight loss obstacles before getting started. Is it a bad knee? Exercise or recuperate.

Veggie aversion? Add a new vegetable to your diet each week. This will slowly help your taste buds get new flavors.

Soda addiction? Start replacing your soda and carbonated drinks with water and mineral drinks.

DO NOT BE IN A RUSH TO SEE RESULTS.

I repeat, be patient enough and satisfied with every little improvement. Rome is not built in a day. You might be eating right and exercising appropriately, but there seem to be nothing happening. This is not in any way a fault from you nor the diet, but assuredly, I can say that the alkaline diet, when you stick to it consistently, including exercise, you can lose weight.

However, if after a couple of months, there seem to be no effect still, it is advised that you see your doctor, he/she can be of great help.

To help you work well on your set goal, keep a food diary. In this diary, record everything you put into your mouth. This helps you stay conscious and committed in the process. Once you remember you have to write down everything you eat, including the junks and snack, you will cut down on them and then get used to the exclusion over time. This diary can also be a plain sheet placed on your refrigerator, where you write down everything you have taken to eat.

Most of the times, the reasons people get swayed from their goal of losing weight can be challenges such as:

- Chronic back, neck, or knee problems

- Chronic pain

- Fatigue

Get rid of these obstacles by consulting your doctor. It can be really challenging to exercise with pains and fatigue.

Also, certain people should always consult with a doctor before attempting to cut calories or lose weight, including:

- Children and the elderly

- Pregnant or nursing women

- Person with a chronic illness of any kind

- A person recovering from an illness or surgery

Finally, ask your doctor if physical therapy would be of benefit to you. A physical therapist is one who can help you develop a safe exercise program.

CHAPTER 13

FREQUENTLY ASKED QUESTIONS ABOUT THE ALKALINE DIET

The knowledge about the alkaline diet is relatively new and has been questioned by so many. It seems everybody is excited about the alkaline diet and wants to give it a try, but on the other hand, there seem to be uncertainties about its functions and benefits. Some people have said it is unscientific and can in no way use diet to change the body's pH. You do not want to remain uncertain and ignorant, so keep reading this. It was specially written for you.

It's not news that the alkaline diet is said to help combat certain diseases and health conditions such as Cancer and also normalizing the body to the best pH, which is slightly alkaline. According to the principle guiding the acid-alkaline diet, more acidic foods signifies a more acidic environment in the body while alkalizing foods will have an alkalizing effect on the body and its pH. We would be addressing certain myths about the alkaline diet and correcting your notion about them in this book. Remember that the key and essential point is balance.

From the previous few chapters, we have discussed that acid-forming foods are those food items that when consumed and digested, upon metabolism they leave behind residues of ash that makes the body acidic and in the same vein, alkaline diet alkalizes the body in a similar mechanism. From the superfood list chapter, we have been able to exhaustively mention most of the food, their class that is whether they are acid-forming or alkaline-forming. Keep at your pace and understand that the alkaline diet advocates for a change of eating lifestyle, not forcefully. Slowly and with exposure, you are shown the best in the alkaline diet.

We might want to know what foods are and why they are so important in our life, health, and wellbeing because this knowledge will serve as the bedrock upon which other facts and points will be based. We do know that human existence is hinged on feeding and feeding well. The longest a man can survive without food is about a month, after which death or illnesses will set in. Also, medically, certain foods and diet have been attributed to be the cause of many diseases and ailments such as an excess glucose causing Diabetes, excess fats and oils giving rise to weight gain and obesity, foods not rich in minerals and vitamins being the cause of both mild problems such as eye defects and the chronic ones. If food is that important to living and health, and an alteration can either make or mar your health, then it is expedient to eat what is healthy in order to live and remain healthy.

What do foods generally do? They form the basis of our lives. It is upon these basic forms that life is hinged. Similarly, when you feed on foods high in acid, you give acidic basics to your body, whereas, the body's normal and expected pH should be slightly alkaline. In this condition, the body works best and is healthy. Therefore, eating a diet that is rich in alkaline-forming foods can play a significant role in bringing the body's pH level down to normality (that is, a healthier state of wellbeing), by neutralizing the excess acid present in the body. At a reduced amount of the acid present in the body, there is aa relative decrease in the rate and levels of inflammation, which is the basis for almost all chronic diseases today. It is, therefore, true that the alkaline diet is healthy and capable of neutralizing acids in the body and giving impressive health results. From herbs, vegetables, fresh foods and fruits, essential nutrients, phytochemicals, and minerals in their right and undiluted proportion is provided. What nature gives cannot be undermined. They are the building block and prototype for existence. All materials, foods, and product there ever are, when degraded, they have basic elements in them. These elements, such as Carbon, Oxygen, and Hydrogen are deposited into the body, and they are the fundamental unit life. They are responsible for life processes and metabolism in the body. From the start of this book, we made it clear that pH is the measure of the Hydrogen ions in a fluid or liquid. If the same Hydrogen exists in foods we take, don't you think a slight increase or decrease in the level could occur due to more or less intake, respectively?

How about acid reflux? There exists a connection between the alkaline food you consume and the amount of stomach acid that could cause acid reflux. The alkaline diet prevents and reduces symptoms of acid reflux. The more alkaline-forming foods you consume, the less your chance of having digestion issues is, which could further lead to the acid reflux. Alkaline water is also recommended as an excellent way to stop acid reflux before it even happens.

Some even claim that the alkaline diet helps gout, how true? You should know that Uric acid and its buildup is responsible for the health condition called gout. So, by consuming alkaline-forming foods, the level of uric acid in your body is lowered, and hence, a gout attack is prevented. Certain foods are tagged as "gout triggers," and close observation of the list reveals that they are acid-forming foods, but on the other hand, if you have ever looked at the 'special diet' for gout, you would realize the most of the list are alkaline-forming foods. It is, therefore, indisputable that the alkaline diet can help prevent gout by neutralizing the triggers which are acid-forming foods.

Alkaline diet and allergies seem to be two different lines that are parallel and can never meet, but the alkaline diet has been testified to have reduced allergies in individuals. This can be associated with the fact that allergies are the body's action against whatever is acidic to it. Their symptoms, therefore, subsides when the alkaline diet is followed well and circumspectly. These allergies include but are not restricted to pet dander, pollen, and dust.

Will the alkaline diet prevent Cancer? The emphatic truth is that Cancer cannot survive in an alkaline environment. Cancer works best by creating a conducive environment for itself; this is so that it can grow well and thrive, which is acidic, and consuming excessive acid-forming food is aiding the devil's work. Therefore, by eating an alkaline-rich diet, you tend to create an unconducive environment for Cancer. It is no myth than to say the alkaline diet is an excellent treatment for Cancer.

Oh, yeah! Diabetes has your blood sugar level beyond the norm, and this is due to the consumption of excessive acid-forming foods, but the alkaline diet keeps your blood sugar in check and under control. Acid-forming foods are known to be super high in sugar and glucose level, and they consequently, elevates the blood sugar level.

It's been said too that an acid-forming diet does not demineralize bones and therefore makes the alkaline diet fact flawed and baseless but the alkaline diet advocates that an excessive overtime consumption of acid-forming foods contributes gradually to the deterioration of the body's internal setup. As much as the kidney is an important part of the body system and is known for pH balance and homeostasis, overworking this organ by consuming excessive acid-forming foods will make it less functional, and the pH of the body will then be altered.

From all being said, you can see that myths about the alkaline diet are just myths and no more. The alkaline diet is super useful and efficient. It gives the opportunity to get the best out of nature, eat healthy and fresh foods and fruits, preventing health conditions that are sickly and cures most of them. The benefits of the alkaline diet cannot be overemphasized, but a trial will definitely convince you.

CHAPTER 14

HOW TO IMPLEMENT THE ALKALINE DIET AS A LIFESTYLE FOR LONG TERM BENEFITS.

In this chapter, we will examine some menu lists across the globe in a bid to explain how to maintain balance even with obstacles. The obstacles here mean the daily routine and other affective human relations that could cause hindrance to maintain a good pH level and a healthy lifestyle. This is about how you might be worried about your health status, considering the fact that you are eating foods that are harmful to your health because you are always busy at work. Don't worry, follow this chapter to the end!

EATING OUT

In your daily routine and relationships, you have to understand many things might work against your way to achieving a healthy lifestyle and balancing your pH level. It will look as if you're working so hard, but all to no avail. The truth is life activities will never stop because of you or for your reason to maintain a balanced pH level. For this reason, you might be left with the only option of eating out at a restaurant. Amazingly, the acid of the alkaline diet has diverse flexibility of application so that you wouldn't need to always keep in mind all the morsels of food you take or the number of drinks you have. You have to be careful when you go to the restaurant to eat –most of these people flaunt their vegetables and meat to thrill you. This is because many of their menu lists might not be favorable to you. You have to understand the good ones for you. Regardless, how loving a food class is to you, consider your pH level and the risk in consuming it. In this chapter, you will learn the breakdown of the codes in any restaurant. This is important because you need to maintain a pH and a healthy life. After this chapter, you should be able to do your daily activities, maintain your pH level, and still keep up with the knowledge of the ordering protocols in the restaurant.

CHOOSE THE STYLE OF YOUR DINING

The types of dining and the services providers of a restaurant contribute to the kind of service you get from them. These determiners are done apart from the fare and price of each food item selected. Understanding the variations in the style of the restaurant will guarantee how you would relate with them in maintaining a healthy life and balance pH level. Below are a few types of establishments and the kind of services provided;

Connoisseur: This type of establishment is usually head by a professional chef. It is charming, bright, and great, but the price is always expensive. The chefs will cook the meal for you and cheerfully set it on your table. This kind of restaurant is usually rated on five stars, among others. However, their menu list might be limited based on the understanding of the chef.

Family-size dining: These are usually controlled by a big franchise company. Their menu list always on top and they host a mob of people at once. Although they could very large in size, they permit exchanging of food –even when the person has requested.

Fast-casual: This kind of restaurant is the commonest. It is common because it is more like the traditional style in which people sit at the table and are served accordingly. This is like a fast-food establishment. However, the menu list is not that standard as it is similar to the one used in a joint establishment.

Fast Food: This kind of establishment works in this way; people troop in to eat by making a simple and receiving order. The menu list is very simple and short. This includes a burger, fries, etc. In actuality, a good menu list healthy and alkaline diet are on the casual and Connoisseur establishments. Though the money spent on these is much, the attendants their know-how to manipulate food menu based on their acid-forming level that will suit their customers. Most times, when you eat out, consider eating some delicious meal in the cuisines which will enhance the pH level such as these;

American cuisine: This kind of cuisine has meat, pizza, and things assorted in them like beef, dairy, and fries. You don't have to choose acidic food item such as seafood rather, make your choice within the superfood list mentioned before. You could find varieties of salad here too. Make sure you make the best out of it and still maintain a healthy lifestyle and pH level.

Chinese food: The menu list here are fried foods, and pounded rice. Additionally, you can add egg and vegetables to your choice if you wish to dice it. It is important to abstain from white rice in order not to take in many acids –which is what you are preventing –no matter how it is prepared.

Greek and Mediterranean cuisine: One advantage of this cuisine is that you have the opportunity to take alkalized vegetables and fruits. Other things you can enjoy are chicken shish kebab garnished with pepper –even vegetables –wild rice, grilled chicken, and shrimp that is boiled. You can eat these kinds of food once in a while but do not make it a habit as these foods if consumed regularly, might increase acidity in your body. Do not eat soft bread, pastries from cheese, and lots more. To take one of the best alkalizing dishes, take bulgur and zucchini.

Italian cuisine: If you are around Italian people, most of their restaurants love to use pasta. Note that very many of these are acidic to your pH level. Therefore, try to choose farro pasta. These ones are good for maintaining a healthy lifestyle. You could take pesto garlic or tomatoes too; they are good alkalizing food items. If you would love to take parmesan food, don't take it with any bread products to refrain from acid-forming food.

Japanese food: One thing you enjoy here that maintains lifestyle and pH level is the seaweed. They are a key source of alkaline diets. You could ask for sashimi, fried foods, sushi fish, and lots more. In fact, you start your meal with either vegetable or fish foods. They are very rich in alkalinity for your body.

Mexican food: Do you find yourself around Mexico? Then, you would need to be very careful as most of their restaurant have not been saturated with much of the westernized food. In fact, most of their menu list is around corn –both the tortillas and tamales. You could choose to eat fajitas too as they are a good source of alkaline. They are either with chicken, vegetables or meat. Meanwhile, many of these restaurants have fruits too. You can take many of them.

Thai and Southeast Asian foods: In these establishments, their menu list comprises of foods that are rich in pH level. However, they maintain that richness if one could abstain from the fried foods. Other food items in these restaurants are cabbage, garlic, seaweed soup, garnished fish and chicken and lots more. There are lots of spicy foods in these establishments. You could decide to take a got a good percentage of dairy foods. Just make sure you don't go beyond the pH level for maintaining and healthy lifestyle food ingredients.

CONSUMING WISELY

The last thing to consider is the way you consume food. A typical example is alcohol consumption. Do you feel like taking alcohol yet want to maintain a good pH level and a healthy lifestyle? If you are thinking of taking alcohol, consider taking very little red wine. Although alcohols are not really harmful to your pH level, the processes involved in making them. Based on the fermentation and other processes, it would be advisable to avoid consumption of alcohol –you have to consume wisely. According to findings, people that consume a little amount of red wine are healthier and without any form of an increase in pH level. To balance your pH level and maintain a healthy lifestyle, you must consume wisely and consider the kind of food you eat –even though you may eat out.

CONCLUSION

It has been a long way till here. The summary of all that has been said properly is that the acid-alkaline diet is the greatest way to live life optimally, detoxifying the body, and nourishing the body in return. Consuming alkaline-forming foods ensures that you are on your body's optimal average which is the pH of 7.3

All you need to do is start easy, slow, and steady. Take just a step at a time, one day at a time. With small but consistent changes, you are on your path to healthy living and optimum balance. Being healthy is supposed to fit your lifestyle; you are not put under constraints. İt is flexible and just amazingly great. Just be you throughout the whole process.

It is important to note that to and keep being alkaline, you have to keep being hydrated from time to time. Dehydration has a huge impact on the quality of one's health. Drink water often and always, when you are properly hydrated, a massive difference in what you'd noticed in your body system. Consume a lot of alkaline-forming foods, all of which has been listed and explained in this book. Make sure to be dynamic with them. Acid-forming foods are those you already know are bad for you and them include refined foods, fast foods, chips, ice cream, trans-fats, meat, caffeine, white bread, white pasta and rice, alcohol, dairy, sugar, chocolate, and pizza. It is also comprehensively marked and detailed that when choosing the food for your diet, be sure to work with the ratio 80/20, that is, consume 80 percent alkaline foods and 20 percent acidic foods.

Learn to breathe well and deep too. Oxygen is important in transporting toxins and disposing them away from the body. Remember that most the acids in the body are expelled in the form of carbon dioxide, and this is gotten rid of when you breathe.

Supplements are not left out, which particular supplement to take can be a confusing part of the alkaline diet, but a few have been suggested in this book of which are:

- Green powder

- Alkaline water

- Alkaline minerals

- Omega oils

One more amazing thing about the alkaline diet is that you can do it for life. Unlike other diets, it does not have an expiring date, it is a lifestyle.

This acid-alkaline diet can help preserve muscle mass as you age. It also protects against diabetes.

The alkaline diet is in a way or two similar to some diets and eating habits, but of them all, the alkaline diet stands strong and the best. A list of these similar diets is provided below:

WHOLE-FOOD, PLANT-BASED DIET: this diet is said to be similar to the Acid-Alkaline diet. It is an eating plan that includes lots of veggies, grains, legumes, and fruits. It does not permit processed foods, like the acid-alkaline diet. It is otherwise tagged a vegetarian diet.

FLEXITARIAN DIET: This is plant-based foods but allows for occasional allowances of foods that are not typically considered vegetarian. It is otherwise called a Flexible vegetarian diet. It combines fresh foods and a little bit of other processed and preserved foods.

MEDITERRANEAN DIET: this is also a diet type that encourages one to consume plant-based foods. (This seems to be a common trait of all healthy eating types, right?) The dividing line between the Mediterranean diet and the Alkaline diet is that it allows and encourages its participants to consume fish and chicken. Dairy products such as eggs, milk, etc., are also promoted as good sources of proteins and cell building units.

To go chapter by chapter key summary,

Chapter one discussed what pH value is all about and why you need to know about it. We went through the scaling values of alkaline and how to test for pH level. We also checked through the benefit of alkalinity in the body

The following chapter unravels what alkaline diet is and how it is nutritious to the body. Chiefly in chapter two, we examined the food to eat and those to be careful to consume at a relatively low rate. We as well check through the popular 80/20 rule. Everything is geared towards providing adequate explanations to what alkaline diet is all about.

In chapter three, everything is all about the alkaline diet superfood list. This list was strategically explained in a way to show these foods' pH level in order to provide guidance to attaining optimum health status. The list of foods is typically given to guide you through the types of food to be consumed. Different classes of foods were discussed too. Special attention was drawn to taking alkalizing water and the reason for doing this.

Moving towards chapter four, we discussed how acidity affects the body. To do this, we explained the means of knowing whether a food is acidic or full of alkaline.

After explaining this, we moved to how the western diet has been making us sick. We also explained why people consume them and the primary things to be done to them. Proper attention is paid to what the western diet is and obesity and diabetes.

In chapter six, we examined the herbs and supplements that are alkalizing. To give them a proper explanation, we explained how to maintain and enhance alkalize diet in the body. Every herbs and supplement explained in the line of how to keep a good alkalizing body.

The following chapter discussed some health conditions that could be improved by the alkaline diet. This was explained in line with how some conditions relating the part of the body that could be cured using the alkaline diet.

In chapter eight, we examined the acidic effect of stress, anger, and negative thinking on mental health, physical health and consequently, the totality of optimum health status. We also explained how some psychological stuff could harm the general optimum health status of the body.

As we moved ahead, we checked through how to maintain high energy using the alkaline diet. This alongside the fact that the alkaline diet is of great importance is the fact that we will need it to carry out adequate body metabolism.

Aside from your devotion to eating what is right, you have learned in chapter ten that your workout can be a factor contributing to the build-up of acids in your system. Not all workouts support and promote alkalinity. The workouts that promote alkalinity are aerobics that builds cardio and controlled breathing. These aerobics increase the flow of oxygen to the heart, muscles, lungs, blood, and cells. This flow helps to detoxify the tissues and provide the necessary circulation of nutrients by the help of oxygen.

Then in chapter eleven we examined the traditional fasting methods and what scientists have to say about it. Then, we unraveled a particularly important method which is intermittent fasting on the Alkaline diet. This fasting, though practiced by many people, unknowingly remains an essential part of maintaining a good pH level, and detoxifying the body. All the times that intermittent fasting covers were duly explained, then we explained how intermittent fasting might have different effects on women than on men, and we gave women the solution to make the most out of intermittent fasting.

In chapter twelve, we explained the pitfalls in weight loss and how you should be able to determine the kind of food to eat and what degree some others are needful in the body in order to achieve optimum balance and health.

Moving towards the end of the book, we answered some frequently asked questions about the alkaline diet.

In the last chapter, we explained how to balance daily routines with the pH level such that none is affecting each other. Everything was explained in order to give the analysis of maintaining optimum health status.

I am sure that your desired and heartfelt questions have been answered and you now know better. If you still have any questions this book did not answer, please do not hesitate to ask us at healthyishfix.com and we will make sure you get the guidance and information you are looking for.

You have been presented with the right knowledge in this book, and your perspective about food and nutrition have been hopefully changed for the better. Acidic foods are not condemned either is alkaline made the hero of the day. But the right meal at the right time in the right way and proportion is the key. Acid-forming foods are good, but alkaline foods are better. But the Acid-Alkaline balanced Food is the King of health, weight loss, energy retention, preventive and curative measures to diabetes, being overweight, having high blood pressure, struggling with chronic fatigue and stress, acne, acid reflux, depressions, inflammations, to mention but a few.

After the whole process as a beginner, your taste buds will change, and you become one who is in love with nutrient-rich food. Hence, your formal junky life where you visit just any restaurant and eat just anything place in front of you changes. You are more conscious about what you eat and how to achieve maximum health.

By now, you know that the Acid-Alkaline diet is not a rigid one but the obvious changes you will experience when you are following this diet is when you stick to it from start to finish. That is, from whenever it is you start till you are transformed and can eat the acid-alkaline diet effortlessly.

REFERENCES

Abelow B. Understanding Acid-Base. New York: Lippincott williams & Wilkins; 1998

Alkaline Herbal Medicine

Aqiyl A. Alkaline Herbal Medicine. 2016

Christopher Vasey. Acid-Alkaline foods chart

Christopher Vasey. The Acid-Alkaline Diet for Optimum Health

Gene Bruno. Acid-Alkaline Balance and Health: An Examination of the Data. 2013

Julie R. And Brown S. Acid-Alkaline Balance and Its Effect on Bone Health. Intl J Integrative Med 2000

Julie w. Acid Alkaline Diet for Dummies. 2013

The Joy of Food: The alkaline way guide. Health Studies Collegium

https://yurielkaim.com/highly-alkaline-foods/

https://m.food24.com/News-and-Guides/Food-in-Focus/10-amazing-recipes-charged-with-high-alkaline-foods-20160518

https://m.food24.com/News-and-Guides/Food-in-Focus/10-amazing-recipes-charged-with-high-alkaline-foods-20160518#menu

https://draxe.com/alkaline-diet/

https://www.globalhealingcenter.com/natural-health/intermittent-fasting/amp/

https://www.dummies.com/food-drink/special-diets/acid-alkaline-diet-for-dummies-cheat-sheet/

https://www.healthline.com/nutrition/intermittent-fasting-for-women#best-types-for-women

www.ingramcontent.com/pod-product-compliance
Lightning Source LLC
Chambersburg PA
CBHW031114250726
48655CB00004B/1709